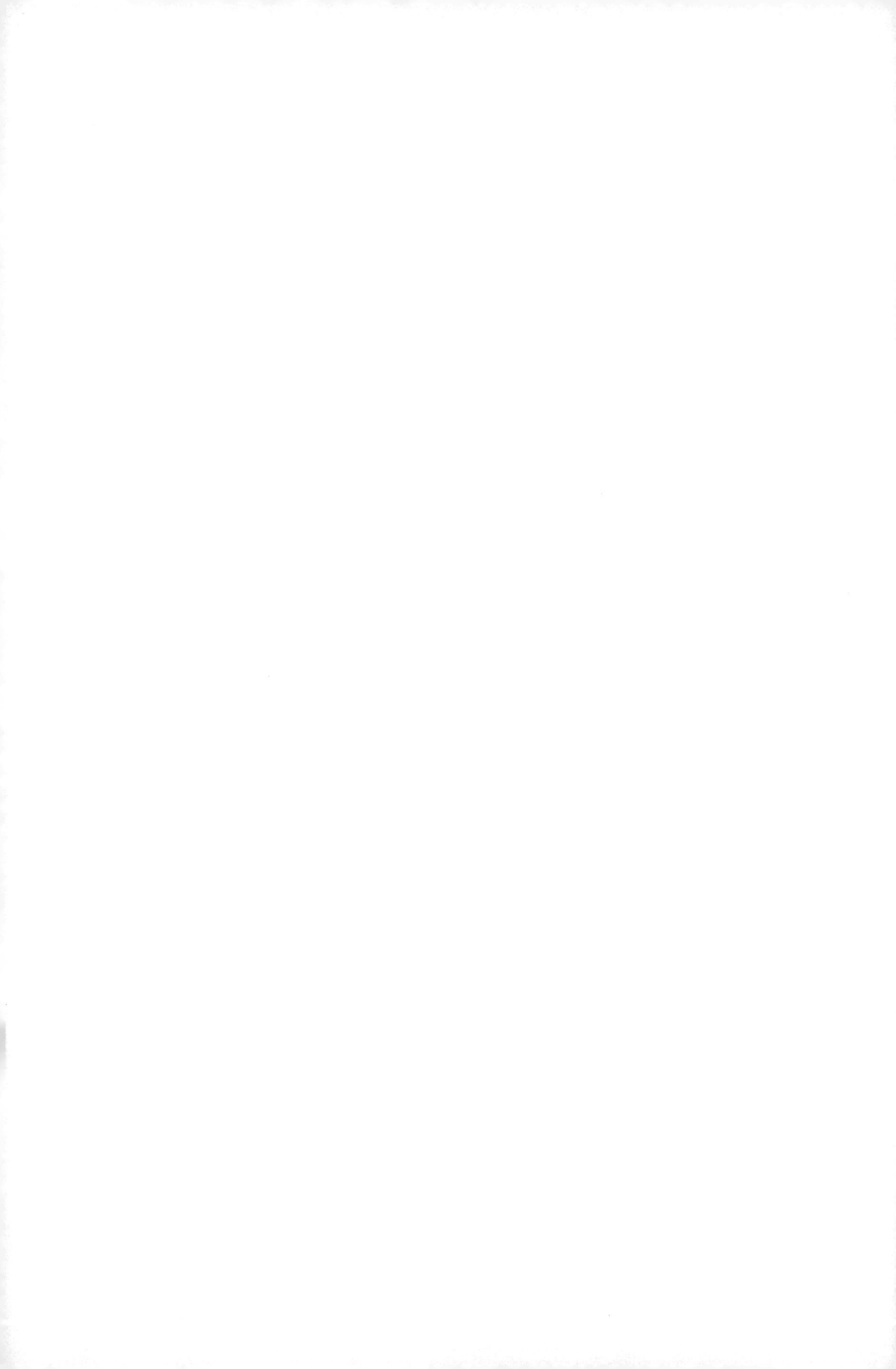

Matthias Alexander Dupuch

Implantable Pressure Sensor Encapsulation for Ventricular Assist Device Control

Matthias Alexander Dupuch

Implantable Pressure Sensor Encapsulation for Ventricular Assist Device Control

Hartung-Gorre Verlag Konstanz

Reprint of Diss. ETH No. 30340

Scientific Reports on Micro and Nanosystems **Volume 38**

edited by Prof. Dr. Christofer Hierold
ETH Zürich
Micro and Nanosystems

Cover images:
Front:

- **Left:** CAD drawing of the implant
- **Middle:** Cross-sectional view of the implant
- **Right:** SEM image of the nanostructured surface

Back:

- **Left:** Etched cannula of the pilot implant
- **Middle:** Photographic and x-ray images of the implant after implantation
- **Right:** Recorded data from animal trial

Bibliographic information published by Die Deutsche Nationalbibliothek

Die Deutsche Nationalbibliothek lists this publication in the Deutsche Nationalbibliografie; detailed bibliographic data is available in the internet at http://dnb.dnb.de.

First edition 2025
HARTUNG-GORRE VERLAG, KONSTANZ
http://www.hartung-gorre.de

ISSN 2566-7769
ISBN 978-3-86628-834-8

DISS. ETH NO. 30340

Implantable Pressure Sensor Encapsulation for Ventricular Assist Device Control

A thesis submitted to attain the degree of

DOCTOR OF SCIENCES
(Dr. sc. ETH Zurich)

presented by

Matthias Alexander Dupuch
MSc. in Micro and Nanosystems, ETH Zurich

born 12.05.1986

accepted on the recommendation of
Prof. Dr. Christofer Hierold
Prof. Dr. Mirko Meboldt
Prof. Dr. Toshiyuki Tsuchiya

2024

"Everything"

- *Thanos*

Dedicated to you, who seeks knowledge on this topic

Abstract

Autonomous feedback controlled ventricular assists device (VAD) operation promises a plethora of benefits such as increased patient safety, comfort, and reduced healthcare costs. Current generation VADs operate at static pump speeds due to the lack of available biocompatible, long-term stable pressure sensor systems.

In this thesis, a pressure sensor encapsulation was developed and integrated in an inflow cannula for a VAD and in an implantable testing platform for animal trials. The encapsulation uses a media separating diaphragm embedded in a Parylene C coating. The approach is expanded to enable optimized diaphragm shapes, which allow significantly better control over the final device characteristics, especially the temperature cross sensitivity. Furthermore, a production processes was developed to minimize assembly induced internal overpressure.

The produced capsules showed excellent pressure transmission of more than 99.7 % and a temperature cross sensitivity of less than 266 Pa from 35 °C to 42 °C for most capsules. However, a large temperature cross sensitivity was observed from room to body temperature in some capsules, adding relevant drift of 750 Pa (75 % quartile) after 42 days to the measurement. The observed drift is related to the viscoelastic nature of the Parylene C diaphragm and the capsule-to-capsule variation is attributed to production process variations, which can be further optimized.

Systematic errors in the pressure transmission, temperature cross sensitivity (TCS), and drift were extracted and correction approaches for each were developed. This enabled the reduction of the pressure transmission error by 50 % by linear correction. A differential measurement approach reduced the temperature cross sensitivity to less than 70 Pa from 35 °C to 42 °C and drastically reduced the temperature induced drift to 300 Pa (75 % quartile) after a jump from room to body temperature. Half of all sensors even remained within a ± 100 Pa window in the same time period.

An alternative drift correction solution was developed based on the Burgers model for viscoelastic materials. This approach performed almost as well as the differential correction, but with the added benefit of being applicable to single sensor systems.

One of the implantable testing platforms was used in three acute animal trials. It matched the systolic and diastolic pressures recorded by a catheter tip sensor within a $\pm$ 133 Pa window for most measurements.

The developed solutions and gained understanding with the proof of concept device build a solid foundation for future pressure sensor integrations for VAD applications.

Zusammenfassung

Der autonome feedback gesteuerte Betrieb von ventrikulaeren unterstuetzungs Pumpen (VAD) verspricht eine Fuelle von Vorteilen wie erhoehte Patientensicherheit, Komfort und reduzierte Gesundheitskosten. VADs der aktuellen Generation operieren aufgrund des Mangels an verfuegbaren biokompatiblen, langzeitstabilen Drucksensorsystemen mit statischen Pumpgeschwindigkeiten.

In dieser Arbeit wurde eine Drucksensorverkapselung entwickelt und in eine Zuflusskanuele fuer ein VAD sowie in eine implantierbare Testplattform fuer Tierversuche integriert. Die Verkapselung verwendet eine medientrennende Membran, die in eine Parylene C-Beschichtung eingebettet ist. Des weiteren wurde dieser Ansatz erweitert, um optimierte Membranformen zu ermoeglichen, was eine deutlich bessere Kontrolle ueber die finalen Geraeteeigenschaften, insbesondere die Temperaturquerempfindlichkeit, ermoeglichen. Darueber hinaus wurde ein Produktionsverfahren entwickelt, um den montagebedingten internen Ueberdruck zu minimieren.

Die hergestellten Kapseln zeigten eine hervorragende Druckuebertragung von mehr als 99,7 % und eine Temperaturquerempfindlichkeit von weniger als 266 Pa von 35 °C bis 42 °C fuer die meisten Kapseln. Allerdings wurde bei einigen Kapseln eine hohe Temperatur-Querempfindlichkeit von Raum- zu Koerpertemperatur beobachtet, welche eine relevante Drift von 750 Pa (75 % Quartil) nach 42 Tagen zur Messung hinzufuegt. Die Drift entspringt der viskoelastischen Natur von Parylene C und die Variation unter den Kapseln ist der Produktionsprozessvariation zuzuordnen, welche weiterer Optimierung bedarf.

Systematische Fehler in der Druckuebertragung, Temperaturquerempfindlichkeit und Drift wurden extrahiert und entsprechende Korrekturansaetze entwickelt. Dadurch konnte der Druckuebertragungsfehler durch lineare Korrektur um 50 % reduziert werden. Ein differenzieller Messansatz reduzierte die Temperaturquerempfindlichkeit auf weniger als 70 Pa von 35 °C auf 42 °C und reduzierte die temperaturinduzierte Drift drastisch auf 300 Pa (75 %-Quartil). Die Haelfte aller Sensoren blieb im gleichen Zeitraum sogar innerhalb eines ± 100 Pa Fensters.

Ein alternativer Drift Korrekturansatz wurde basierend auf dem Burgers Modell fuer viskoelastische Materialien entwickelt. Dieser Ansatz erreichte fast die Qualitaet des differenziellen Messansatzes, bringt aber den Vorteil mit sich, auch bei Systemen mit nur einem Sensor zu funktionieren.

Eine der implantierbaren Testplattformen wurde in drei akuten Tierversuchen verwendet. Sie stimmte bei den meisten Messungen innerhalb eines Fensters von $\pm$ 133 Pa mit den systolischen und diastolischen Druecken ueberein, welche von einem Katheterspitzensensor aufgezeichnet wurden.

Die entwickelten Loesungen und das gewonnene Verstaendnis, zusammen mit dem Proof-of-Concept-Geraet bilden eine solide Grundlage fuer zukuenftige Drucksensorintegrationen in VADs.

Acknowledgements

This work would not have been possible without the help of the many colleagues I have encountered during my time with the Micro and Nanosystems group (MNS). First I would like to thank Prof. Hierold who guided me through this thesis with encouragement, critical questions, and freedom to explore new ideas. Especially his availability for discussions and feedback for options in the planning phase of different subprojects helped plot the course towards meaningful and successful experiments. The frequent interactions with many former and current members of the MNS group have been a fruitful and pleasant experience in which the wide range of professional backgrounds formed a corner stone of this interdisciplinary work.

I would like especially to thank a few people: Dr. Haluska, with whom I had many brainstorming sessions and who helped me through difficult situation already well before the beginning of this project. Dr. Mihailovic and Dr. Nedelcu who helped me cut through electrotechnical problems and who became good friends over the years. Ms. Vehusheia who helped with material-science related questions and was a pleasant office mate. Dr. Jenni who's input in chemical matters often formed the starting point of solutions and my predecessor Dr. Staufert who provided the nanostructure anchoring technology without which the devices produced in this work would not have been realizable. My students Mr. Smesny, Mr. Graf, Mr. Hutter and Mr. Mueller (Pascal) who designed the leak detection setup and tested three components, electrical feedthrough, diaphragm, and backside sealing. Mr. Mueller (Basil) who investigated the nanostructure patterning and Ms. Martin and Ms. Ruth for their efforts towards simulation and experimental understanding of the impact of curvature on the diaphragm. Finally Ms. Kaegi who shielded me from administrative distractions during this project.

Outside of the MNS group, Mr. Willhelm, a former member of the institute for virtual production, who helped accelerate the production process with the fast production of support tools. Dr. Maden of the isotope geochemistry and cosmochemistry group, who provided time, knowledge, expensive equipment and lab space for the helium leak detection tests. Dr. von Petersdorff-Campen from the product development group and our student Mr. Enke with whom we successfully translated the sensor encapsulation to inflow cannulae for a commercial ventricular assist device. I would also thank the Zurich Heart project and its former and current members especially Dr. Cesarovic and Prof. Falk with whom I shared the vision of a next generation ventricular assist device.

Outside of ETH I would like to thank Prof. Starck and his student Mr. Kaemmel who organized and executed the animal trials in this thesis as well as Dr. Unger, Dr. Schmidt and Mr. Bernhard from the veterinarian team.

This work has been supported by the Maexi Stiftung.

List of Abbreviations

Abbreviation	Description
VAD	Ventricular assist device
HF	Heart failure
LVP	Left ventricular pressure
MSD	media separating diaphragm
MSPSE	Media separating pressure sensor encapsulations
TCS	Temperature cross sensitivity
CTE	Coefficient of thermal expansion

List of Symbols

Symbol	Description	S.I. Unit
r	radius of the MSD	m
h	thickness of the MSD	m
z	centre deflection of the MSD	m
E	Young's modulus of the MSD material	Pa
ν	Poisson's ratio of the MSD material	-
V_D	deflection volume of the MSD	m^3
V_L	volume change of the encapsulated liquid	m^3
V_B	volume change of the encapsulated bubble	m^3
c	deflection volume coefficient of the MSD	m
p_{in}	pressure inside the MSPSE	Pa
p_{out}	pressure outside of the MSPSE	Pa
T	temperature	K
k	spring constant	N/m
d	dampening constant	Ns/m

1 mmHg = 1 Torr = 133.322 Pa = 1.33322 mbar

Contents

Abstract iii

Zusammenfassung v

Acknowledgements vii

List of Abbreviations ix

List of Symbols xi

List of Figures xvii

List of Tables xxi

1 Introduction 1
- 1.1 Heart Failure 1
- 1.2 The State of VADs 2
- 1.3 Motivation 2

2 State of the Art 5
- 2.1 Sensor Characterization 5
- 2.2 Bloodpressure Sensing for Application in VADs 5
- 2.3 Cannula Deformation Measurement 9
- 2.4 Sensor Encapsulation 9
- 2.5 Hybrid Approach 10
- 2.6 Summary 10
- 2.7 Related non-Integrated Sensors 10
- 2.8 Summary, Motivation and Objectives 11

3 Pressure Sensor Encapsulation 13
- 3.1 Basic Pressure Sensor Encapsulation 14
  - 3.1.1 Influence on Measured Pressure 14
- 3.2 Pressure Transmission 15
  - 3.2.1 The Media Separating Diaphragm 15
  - 3.2.2 Pressure Transmission Fluid 17
  - 3.2.3 Pressure Transmission Model 19
- 3.3 Temperature Cross Sensitivity 22

3.4 Drift 25
3.5 Viscoelasticity 25
3.5.1 Implications for this Project 27
3.6 Analysis of Previous Demonstrator Device 29
3.6.1 Challenges 30
3.7 MSD Design for Implants 34
3.7.1 Model vs. Reality 36

4 Approach of the Thesis **39**
4.1 Goals 39
4.2 Implantable Testing Platform 40
4.3 MSD 42
4.4 Pressure Transmission Fluid 43
4.5 Electrical Feedthrough 43
4.6 Backside Sealing 44

5 Individual Components **45**
5.1 MSD 46
5.1.1 MSD Shape 46
5.1.2 Materials & Methods 46
5.1.3 Results & Discussion 51
5.1.4 Conclusion 57
5.2 Channel Plug 62
5.2.1 Materials & Methods 62
5.2.2 Results & Discussion 62
5.2.3 Conclusion 64
5.3 Electrical Feedthrough 65
5.3.1 Materials & Methods 65
5.3.2 Results & Discussion 67
5.3.3 Conclusion 69
5.4 Backside Sealing 70
5.4.1 Materials & Methods 72
5.4.2 Results & Discussion 72
5.4.3 Conclusion 72
5.5 Component Leakage 74

6 Implant Characterization **77**
6.1 Pressure Transmission 77
6.1.1 Materials & Methods 77
6.1.2 Results & Discussion 78
6.1.3 Conclusion 80
6.2 Temperature Cross Sensitivity 82
6.2.1 Materials & Methods 82
6.2.2 Results & Discussion 84
6.2.3 Conclusion 86

6.3 Drift 87
6.3.1 Materials & Methods 87
6.3.2 Results & Discussion 88
6.3.3 Conclusion 90

7 Error Reduction for Implants **91**
7.1 Pressure Transmission Correction 91
7.1.1 Materials & Methods 91
7.1.2 Results & Discussion 92
7.1.3 Conclusion 92
7.2 Drift Correction 93
7.2.1 Materials & Methods 95
7.2.2 Results & Discussion 96
7.2.3 Conclusion 98
7.3 Temperature Cross Sensitivity Correction 98
7.3.1 Materials & Methods 98
7.3.2 Results & Discussion 99
7.3.3 Conclusion 100
7.4 Overall Residual Error 100
7.4.1 Suggested approach 102

8 Model Based TCS Correction **105**
8.1 Burgers Model Based Correction 105
8.1.1 Materials & Methods 107
8.1.2 Results & Discussion 110
8.1.3 Conclusion 118

9 In-Vivo Experiment **121**
9.1 Animal Trial with Catheter Tip Pressure Sensor Reference . . 121
9.1.1 Materials & Methods 122
9.1.2 Results & Discussion 123
9.1.3 Conclusion 125

10 Conclusion and Outlook **127**
10.1 Summary & Accomplishments 127
10.2 Discussion & Outlook 129

11 List of Student Projects **131**

12 List of Publications **133**
12.0.1 Article 133
12.0.2 Oral Abstract 133

Curriculum Vitae **135**

A Appendix A **137**
A.1 Implant Characterization 137
A.2 Error Correction 142
A.3 Model Based TCS Correction (Burgers Model) 147
A.4 Animal Trial (ch. 8) 151

Bibliography **155**

List of Figures

3.1 Schematic: Typical pressure sensor encapsulation 14
3.2 Schematic: Small vs. large deflection 15
3.3 Schematic: MSPSE, deflection and bubble compression 19
3.4 Calc: MSD deflection vs. bubble compression 20
3.5 Calc: Parameter variation and pressure transmission 21
3.6 Calc: TCS for enclosed air content 23
3.7 Calc: Parameter variation and TCS 24
3.8 Schematic: Drift types 25
3.9 Schematic: Burgers model 26
3.10 Calc: Viscoelastic material and time 27
3.11 Calc: Viscoelastic stress-strain loop 28
3.12 Schematic: Previous demonstrator device, cross-section 29
3.13 Calc: TCS for enclosed air content, prev. demo. device . . . 31
3.14 Calc: Assembly process, prev. demo. device 32
3.15 Schematic: Observed wax-plug failure modes 32
3.16 Calc: Pressure sensitivity during assembly, prev. demo. device 33
3.17 Schematic: Pill-shaped curved MSD 34
3.18 Calc: TCS, pill-shaped MSD 36
3.19 Calc: Pressure transmission, pill-shaped MSD 37

4.1 CAD: Exploded view of the implant 40
4.2 CAD: Cross section of MSPSE in implant 41
4.3 Schematic: Layout of the sensor readout electronics system . 42

5.1 Flowchart: MSPSE production overview 45
5.2 Schematic: MSD shaping process 47
5.3 Photo: Photolithography for MSD shaping 50
5.4 SEM: Nanostructures 52
5.5 Photo: Wax disc shaping 53
5.6 Result: Wax disc thickness histogram 53
5.7 WLI: Wax disc surface profile 54
5.8 Photo: MSD from cured/uncured wax disc 55
5.9 SEM: Etch border region 56
5.10 Result: Etch depth vs time 57
5.11 Results: Etch time and depth distribution 58
5.12 Photo: Half cleaned MSD bed 59

5.13 Photo: Etched pill-shaped MSD bed 60
5.14 Photo: Wax patch vs. etch route result 61
5.15 Schematic: Sugar plug process 62
5.16 Photo: Sugar plug formation 63
5.17 Photo: Sugar plug in implant 64
5.18 WLI: Surface profile of a sugar plug 65
5.19 CAD: Electrical feedthrough 66
5.20 Schematic: Electrical feedthrough fabrication 67
5.21 Photo: Implant solder Jig 68
5.22 Photo: Metallized implant 69
5.23 Photo: Electrical feedthrough assembly 70
5.24 Schematic: Oilfill and backside sealing process 71
5.25 Photo: Backside sealing cross-section 73
5.26 Data: Pressure during backside sealing 74

6.1 Schematic: Pressure testing station 78
6.2 Data: Pressure transmission test protocol 79
6.3 Data: Pressure transmission error, implants 80
6.4 Data: Pressure transmission error relative, implants 81
6.5 Calc: Pressure transmission, pill-shaped MSD, var fill-pres. . 81
6.6 Data: TCS test protocol for operating range 83
6.7 Data: Pressure transmission test protocol 83
6.8 Data: TCS in operating range, implants 84
6.9 Data: Measured vs calculated TCS 85
6.10 Data: Initial pressure jump 85
6.11 Data: Initial pressure jump evolution 86
6.12 Data: Drift measurement protocol 87
6.13 Data: Drift measurement 33 d 88
6.14 Data: Drift vs initial increase 89
6.15 Data: Iterative and total drift 90

7.1 Data: Pressure transmission error after correction 92
7.2 Schematic: Schematic of a reference capsule 93
7.3 Data: Drift correction process 95
7.4 Data: Drift error after correction 96
7.5 Data: Implantwise drift error after correction 97
7.6 Data: TCS after drift correction 99
7.7 Data: Error window after correction 101
7.8 Data: Error source comparison 101

8.1 Schematic: Burgers Model as used 105
8.2 Data: Linearization of temperature pressure relation 108
8.3 Flowchart: Burgers model parameter fitting 109
8.4 Data: Example of Burgers model solutions, 4th Run, 1/1/1 . 112

8.5 Data: Example of Burgers model solutions, 4th Run, 1/1/1, zoom . . . 113
8.6 Data: Example of Burgers model solutions, 4th Run, 1/2/1 . 114
8.7 Data: Example of Burgers model solutions, 4th Run, 1/2/1, zoom . . . 115
8.8 Data: Example of Burgers model solutions, 5th Run, 1/1/1 . 116
8.9 Data: Example of Burgers model solutions, 5th Run, 1/2/1 . 117
8.10 Data: Residual errors after model based correction, zoom . . 118

9.1 Photo: Implantation . . . 122
9.2 Data: Animal trial pressure curve . . . 123
9.3 Data: Systolic and diastolic deviation . . . 124
9.4 Data: Internal Systolic and diastolic deviation . . . 125

A.1 Photo: Pressure testing station . . . 138
A.2 Data: Drift measurement run 1 . . . 138
A.3 Data: Drift measurement run 2 . . . 139
A.4 Data: Drift measurement run 3 . . . 139
A.5 Data: Drift measurement run 5 . . . 140
A.6 Data: Drift vs initial increase . . . 140
A.7 Data: Drift vs initial increase . . . 141
A.8 Data: Drift vs initial increase . . . 141
A.9 Data: Drift vs initial increase . . . 142
A.10 Data: Drift error after correction zoomed out . . . 143
A.11 Data: Implantwise drift error projection . . . 144
A.12 Data: Error window projection 3m . . . 144
A.13 Data: Error contribution proj. 3m . . . 145
A.14 Data: Error window projection 1y . . . 145
A.15 Data: Error contribution proj. 1y . . . 146
A.16 Data: Residual errors after model based correction, zoom . . 148
A.17 Data: Residual errors after model based correction, 121J4 . . 149
A.18 Data: Residual errors after model based correction, 121J4 . . 149
A.19 Data: Linear calibration data of the 4th animal trial . . . 151
A.20 Data: Linear calibration parameters of the 4th animal trial . 151
A.21 Data: Raw recorded data of the 4th animal trial . . . 152

List of Tables

2.1 Sensor characterization 6
2.2 Literature 1/2 7
2.3 Literature 2/2 8

3.1 Pill-shaped MSD parameters 36

5.1 Samples and process route 46

7.1 Error projection classification 102

8.1 Burges parameter compare 107
8.2 List of req. for both correction approaches 118

A.1 List of req. for both correction approaches 137
A.2 k and d values for 1/2/1 150
A.3 List of animal trials. 153

1 Introduction

Ventricular assist devices (VADs) are mechanical pumps that suck the blood out of the heart and inject it into the Aorta. They are implanted in patients with end-stage heart failure (HF), a condition where the heart is unable to supply sufficient blood flow to the body. Current generation VADs are unable to autonomously adjust to the body's needs, which can lead to severe complications, some of which can be life threatening.

1.1 Heart Failure

Heart failure (HF) is the inability of the heart to sufficiently perfuse body and organs with blood and one of the world's leading cause of hospitalization and death [1]. HF is affecting 40 million people or around 2 % of the population world-wide [1–3]. These numbers are expected to increase by 46 % in the next decade for the U.S., where the probability of HF triples with every decade lived above 60 and around half of all patients diagnosed with HF die within 5 years [3].

The stage of HF can be classified by the ejection fraction, the volume of blood pumped per stroke by the patient, compared to that of a healthy person. In its early stages, HF often remains unnoticed by the patient but requires medical treatment once it progresses. In its final stage, a transplant or mechanical support becomes mandatory for survival [1,3].

While heart transplantation remains the gold standard, the shortage of donor hearts dictates the selection of alternative treatment routes [4, 5]. Current third generation VADs are implantable, transportable, continuous-flow, turbo dynamic pumps that support the function of the heart without replacing it [4]. In the case of left VADs the pump sucks blood out of the left ventricle and injects it into the aorta via bypass graft. In this manner, the reduced pumping activity of the heart is compensated, and perfusion of the body is restored. These pumps are becoming an increasingly viable option, not only as "bridge-to-transplant" but also for recovery and as a definite treatment option with 2 year survival rates reaching 70 % and 40 % after 5 years [6].

1.2 The State of VADs

While offering a new path forward when no donor heart was available, first generation VADs still suffered from mechanical reliability issues and multiple medical complications such as thrombus formation, non-surgical bleeding, strokes, and hemolysis [4]. With the second generation of VADs, mechanical reliability was significantly improved, even exceeding the expected service duration. However, the medical complications remained. Third generation VADs, were designed with durability and improved hemocompatibility in mind [4]. The later promising a reduction in adverse events resulting directly from the induced blood trauma, and therefore also a reduction of the necessary blood trauma medication and its side effects [4].

Additional harm can be inflicted on the patient when the pump speed does not meet the current, ever changing, requirements of the human body. Under- and over pumping can lead to impaired right heart function, arrhythmia, pulmonary edema, ischemia of the heart and other organs, hemolysis, thrombogenesis, strokes, suction events, tissue damage, ventricle collapse, and death [5, 7–9]. Currently, the pump speed is fixed post-implantation by a physician under echocardiographic monitoring and some VADs further give limited influence over the speed in form of predefined modes for the patient to switch manually [10]. Some VADs offer suction event detection, based on flow measurements and sudden changes of the rotor operation behaviour to temporarily reduce the pump speed. Besides that, the flow is only passively and insufficiently adjusted around the set fixed pump speed, by the pre- and afterload sensitivity inherent to any pump system [4, 5].

An additional concern is the reduced or absent pulsatility which originates from the continuos-flow operation of turbo dynamic VADs. It has been suggested to cause increased incident rates of multiple organ dysfunction syndrome and gastrointestinal bleeding [10, 11].

1.3 Motivation

Feedback control of the VAD promises almost instantaneous and adaptable adjustment of the pump speed to the momentary need of the body, eliminating patient interaction and reducing clinic visits [5]. Precise control over the pump speed can also enable improved treatment methods [12], improved perfusion [13], and even Frank-Starling-like pump behaviour, mimicking the natural pumping response of the heart [5]. Multiple control variables, to be used individually or combined, such as left ventricular pressure (LVP) [14] [15] [16], left arterial pressure, left ventricular volume [17], LVP to volume relationship, aortic pressure [18] [19], heart rate [8] [20], pulsatility index, pulsatility gradient, pulsatility ratio, constant average pressure difference between aorta and left atrium, and constant average differential pump pressure have been suggested for VAD control algorithms [5].

Tchantchaleishvili et al. conclude that LVP is the most suitable control variable for feedback control. The validity of LVP-based control and its superiority over constant speed operation has also been demonstrated in-vitro [21] and tested in-vivo by Petrou et al. [22].

However, the implementation of LVP-based control demands a precise pressure sensor integration solution with high long-term trueness and high hemocompatibility, which is currently unavailable [5].

2 State of the Art

2.1 Sensor Characterization

To characterize the performance of a sensor system three terms are used here: trueness, precision and accuracy. Trueness refers to systematic errors, such as an offset error. Precision refers to random errors, such as noise. Accuracy describes the combination of trueness and precision and thus refers to the total error in the system [23].

2.2 Bloodpressure Sensing for Application in VADs

Multiple approaches for pressure sensing in VADs have been explored and follow two concepts: measurement of the deformation (strain) of the inflow cannula or integration of an encapsulated sensor into the inflow cannula.

In the former category two approaches have been explored. First, local thinning of the cannula wall to create an area which deflects under physiological pressure. Strain gauges, attached to the non-blood-contacting side of that area, were then used to measure the deflection [24, 25]. Stephens et al. followed a more radical approach by replacing the stiff steel with a soft silicone tube. The strain was converted into wavelength shift by Bragg-grating in an optical fibre wrapped around the cannula [26]. This approach brings the advantage of a well-defined, smooth blood contacting surface.

In the latter category, multiple approaches aiming at placing an encapsulated pressure sensor in a cut-out in the side wall of an inflow cannula have been explored [13, 27, 28]. This approach offers the possibility to leverage the full power and experience of the semiconductor pressure sensor industry by biocompatible encapsulation.

Alternatively to the encapsulated sensor, a patterned media separating diaphragm (MSD) was placed in the cut-out and its deformation was measured by Fabry Perot interferometry [29].

A hybrid approach was explored by Staufert at al., where the MSD was integrated as part of a complete coating of a cannula covering a cut-out in its wall. The pressure sensor was then placed in the oil-filled cavity behind the MSD [30]. This combines the advantages of both categories by fully integrating the cannula and its biocompatible coating into the sensor encapsulation concept.

Table 2.1: Typical properties used to characterize sensors and the goals set for this project

<table>
<tr><th>Property</th><th>Description</th><th>Limits</th></tr>
<tr><td>Range</td><td>Capability to record the range of possible pressures</td><td>-2.7 to 24 kPa
p_0 = ambient</td></tr>
<tr><td>Zero error</td><td>Offset error</td><td rowspan="5">Correctable if repeatable</td></tr>
<tr><td>Span error</td><td>Linear deviation proportional to the value change</td></tr>
<tr><td>Pressure non-linearity</td><td>Non-linear deviation to the value change</td></tr>
<tr><td>Thermal effect on zero</td><td>Temperature induced offset error</td></tr>
<tr><td>Thermal effect on span</td><td>Temperature induced span error</td></tr>
<tr><td>Pressure hysteresis</td><td>Pressure induced hysteresis</td><td rowspan="5">Total Error:

Diastole:
$< \pm$ 400 Pa

Systole:
$< \pm$ 800 Pa

until recalibration</td></tr>
<tr><td>Thermal hysteresis</td><td>Temperature induced hysteresis</td></tr>
<tr><td>Ratiometricity</td><td>Influence of supply voltage fluctuation</td></tr>
<tr><td>Drift</td><td>Amalgam of effects altering the signal over time</td></tr>
<tr><td>Non-repeatability</td><td>Other non-repeatable effects, e.g. hysteresis</td></tr>
<tr><td>Response time</td><td>Step response time</td><td>$>$ 11 kPa/0.05 s</td></tr>
</table>

Table 2.2: List of research on sensor systems for pressure sensing in ventricular assist devices (Part 1/2)

Device	Sensor Type	Location	Pressure Sensitivity	Range [mmHg]	Resol. [mmHg]	Offset Drift	Nonlin. [mmHg]
Bullister 2001 [24]	thin-film strain gauge	in/outflow	-	-425 to 300	-	0.4 to 20 mmHg/y (n=2)	0.4 to 0.59 (n=3)
Saito 2008 [13]	Pu MSD piezo resistive	inflow	-	-	-	-	-
Shi 2008 [27]	Pu MSD piezo resistive	inflow	-	ca. 0 to 110	-	24 mmHg/5 m	-
Fritz 2010 [25]	semi-con strain gage	in/outflow	0.52±0.24 µV/mmHg	0 to 75	-	180 and -140 mmHg/4 weeks	-
Zhou 2012 [31]	Fabry Perot interferometer	inflow	-	0 to 180	1	-	-
Brancato 2016 [28]	piezo resistive senso r	outflow	12 µV/V/mmHg	0 to 350	-	first 50h: 8.3 mmHg then: 0.05 mmHg/d	-
Staufert 2016 [30]	piezo resistive sensor	inflow	0.987	-730 to 200	-	Near 0 in 30 d	-
Stephens 2019 [26]	optical wire diffraction	Inflow	-4.4 to -5.1 pm/mmHg	-25 to 250	+/- 0.019	-	-
Dupuch 2021 [46]	piezo resistive sensor	inflow	> 0.99	-100 to 200	-	-	-

Table 2.3: List of research on sensor systems for pressure sensing in ventricular assist devices (Part 2/2)

Device	TCS [mmHg/°C]	Hysteresis [mmHg]	Error [mmHg]	Response Time	in-vivo Accuracy	In-Vivo?
Bullister 2001 [24]	-	0.64 to 0.87 (n=3)	0.45 to 0.87	-	2 to 3 mmHg	acute
Saito 2008 [13]	-	-	-	-	-	chronic 2m
Shi 2008 [27]	-	-	2	-	2 mmHg	chronic 5m
Fritz 2010 [25]	Span: 35 to -41 Gain: -14 to 9.4	15 to 4.1 at 75 mmHg, 4h	-	90 mmHg/2.2 ms	N/A	no
Zhou 2012 [31]	-	-	-	48.5 mmHg/s	N/A	no
Brancato 2016 [28]	Offset: -6% FS Sens.: 0.01% FS	-	-	-	-	acute (awoken)
Staufert 2016 [30]	-	-	-	-	N/A	no
Stephens 2019 [26]	base: 2.1 to 2.6 corr.: 0.06 (35-39°C)	no short-term	-	89.7 mmHg/s	N/A	no
Dupuch 2021 [46]	0.9 to 3.3	-	-	-	N/A	no

2.3 Cannula Deformation Measurement

This category focuses on measuring the deformation of the cannula without needing an additional blood-contacting interface. Bullister et al. reported a strain gauge on thinned cannula approach, where, instead of a round inflow cannula, a version with a flattened side resulting in a D shaped cross section was used to achieve a larger MSD area. Sufficient pressure range, rise time and a low error (< 1 mmHg) but with a large offset drift of up to 20 mmHg/y characterize these devices [24]. How the transition from the D-shaped cross-section to the round part affects the flow was not discussed. Fritz et al.'s similar approach used a circular cross-section, trading geometry for lower MSD area. While these devices also showed excellent rise times, the low range and extreme baseline drift limit application to suction event detection [25]. A slightly different approach is explored by Stephen et al. where the inflow cannula material, typically steel or titanium, is replaced by a softer silicone tube. The strain is then transmitted to an attached strainable fiber Bragg grating. This fiber, when strained, shifts the wavelength of light traveling through it. This system shows sufficient range, excellent resolution, low and correctable temperature cross sensitivity, but a slow rise time of 89.7 mmHg/s [26].

2.4 Sensor Encapsulation

This category offers the possibility to leverage the full power and experience of the semiconductor pressure sensor industry by biocompatible encapsulation. Such an encapsulation is necessary to both protect the sensor from the body and vice versa. Saito et al. and Shi et al. chose a polyurethane MSD for the blood-contacting interface and silicone oil as pressure transmission liquid from the MSD to the sensor. A small range and significant drift (24 mmHg/5 months) seem to limit the clinical use. However, using the sensor purely for Systole/Diastole detection allowed an increase in pumped volume of 15 % compared to the standard operation [13]. Furthermore, an automated recalibration mechanism based on suction events was developed. This recalibration allowed them to operate a sensor driven VAD over the course of 5 months in-vivo [27]. Brancato et al. used a Parylene C sensing interface, coated over a silicone embedded pressure sensor. This system showed sufficient range, low drift after an initial 2-day phase, and was validated in-vivo for 12 h [28].

2.5 Hybrid Approach

The hybrid approach, utilizing a Parylene C sensing interface in a fully integrated encapsulation design, explored by Staufert et al., showed excellent accuracy with negligible error of 0.02 mmHg as well as drift-free behavior over the course of 30 days [30].

2.6 Summary

A set of relevant properties for such a pressure measurement system is given in the Table 2.1. Outside of the inherent sensing system behaviour, the short and long-term interaction with the human body needs to be studied [5]. Multiple sensing implementation approaches have been explored (Tab: 2.2 and Tab: 2.3) and show advantages and challenges. Of these devices only Staufert et al. [30] and Brancato et al. [28] meet the criteria (Tab: 2.1), based on the information provided, which is often incomplete.

2.7 Related non-Integrated Sensors

Few commercial, implantable pressure sensors exist on the market today and have been used in pilot studies to observe VAD functionality and support VAD speed adjustments. One of them (ISSYS, Titan, ISS Inc., Ypsilanti, MI) was implanted in the atria of four patients by Hubbert et al., along with a VAD [32–34]. A clear correlation between pump speed and measured pressure was observed in all patients. Furthermore, an unexpected, sudden increase in mean left atrial pressure, recorded during outpatient treatment, triggered a pump exchange. The explanted pump confirmed the suspicion of pump thrombosis [34]. Further studies based on the CardioMEMS implantable pulmonary artery sensor along with a VAD suggest favorable outcome and fewer hospitalizations. This is attributed to improved treatment based on the additional diagnostic information [35]. However, drift and the complex communication systems required for battery-free operation remain challenges both for periodic and live pump adjustment [5,36].

2.8 Summary, Motivation and Objectives

Automated adaptive VAD operation promises a wide range of benefits over the constant speed operation of current generation VADs. While a wide range of research studies with different control algorithm approaches exist, there is currently no sensor system available which is capable of supporting these solutions, neither in research, nor commercially available. The most progressing approach uses an MSD seamlessly integrated into a polymer, VAD inflow cannula coating, enabling undisturbed blood flow [30].

In the first part of this thesis the concept of a media separated pressure sensor encapsulation is analysed and potential sources of pressure error are described, which become especially relevant with respect to drift in the context of a viscoelastic MSD material. the following questions are addressed:

- Which design parameters are relevant for optimal trueness?
- How can the impact of the manufacturing process on trueness be minimized?
- Which outer influences can affect the trueness during operation?
- How can the impact of these influences on the trueness during operation be minimized?

In the second part a produced implantable testing platform is characterized and compared to the model prediction, and approaches to reduce the systematic error are discussed. The following questions are adressed:

- How does the device behave and how does it compared to the model predictions?
- What are the remaining sources of systematic error?
- Can the systematic error be predicted or otherwise eliminated?

3 Pressure Sensor Encapsulation

The pressure sensing inflow cannulae and implants discussed in this work are functionally, media separating pressure sensor encapsulations (MSPSEs). Such capsules serve the purpose of protecting the encapsulated sensor from the environment while maintaining a mechanical pressure transmission chain from the environment to the sensor.

A colored version of this chapter is available at: https://doi.org/10.3929/ethz-b-000702759

Functionally MSPSEs consist of:

- the media separating diaphragm (MSD), the pressure transmitting, hermetic border between outside and inside of the MSPSE
- the pressure transmitting fluid inside the capsule, which transmits the pressure from the MSD to the sensor
- the housing, the border of the capsule, where no pressure transmission is required
- the electrical feedthrough, which electrically connects the inside of the capsule with the outside
- the backside sealing, which hermetically seals in the pressure transmission liquid after filling

These functional components can be merged or split into any imaginable number of physical components which may have additional functions unrelated to the encapsulation (see ch. 4.2).

3.1 Basic Pressure Sensor Encapsulation

Figure 3.1 shows a common concept of an MSPSE. The MSD separates the fluid, which's pressure is to be measured, from the encapsulated sensor and the pressure transmission liquid. The sensor is electrically connected through the boundaries of the capsule via the electrical feedthrough. Such capsules are commonly filled with the pressure transmission liquid at the end of the assembly process via the filling channel and sealed with a ball sealing. This chapter discusses general considerations necessary for the design of MSPSEs.

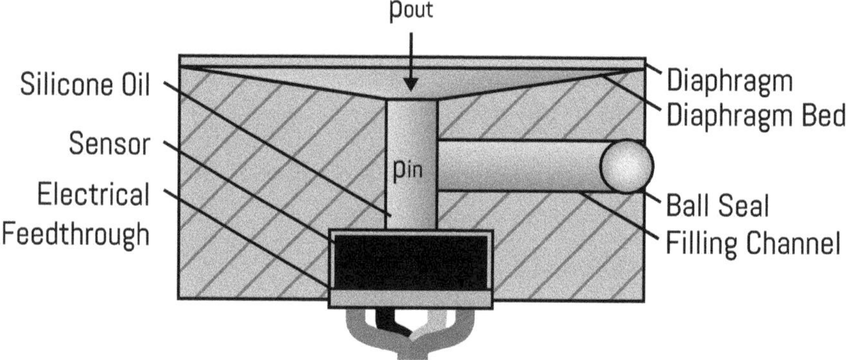

Figure 3.1: Schematic of a typical media-separated pressure sensor encapsulation.

3.1.1 Influence on Measured Pressure

While the encapsulation's purpose is the protection of the sensor, it also affects the measured pressure. Three main effects need to be considered when designing a transmission liquid based encapsulation [37]:

- Pressure transmission
- Temperature cross sensitivity
- Drift

3.2 Pressure Transmission

Pressure transmission describes how well the pressure is transmitted from the outside of the capsule to the sensor inside the capsule.

$$Pressuretransmission = \frac{p_{in} - p_{in}^0}{p_{out} - p_{out}^0} \tag{3.1}$$

where (see fig. 3.1):

- p_{in} is the current pressure inside the capsule,
- p_{out} is the current pressure outside the capsule,
- p_{in}^0 is the initial pressure inside the capsule,
- p_{out}^0 is the initial pressure outside the capsule,

It is governed mainly by the deflection of the MSD and the compression of the pressure transmission fluid.

3.2.1 The Media Separating Diaphragm

At the core of every MSPSE is the MSD, a thin stretchable and bendable sheet. Its deformation under external forces is called deflection. The deflection is the result of the equilibrium between the external forces, caused by a pressure difference across the sheet, and the reactive, internal forces resisting the deformation.

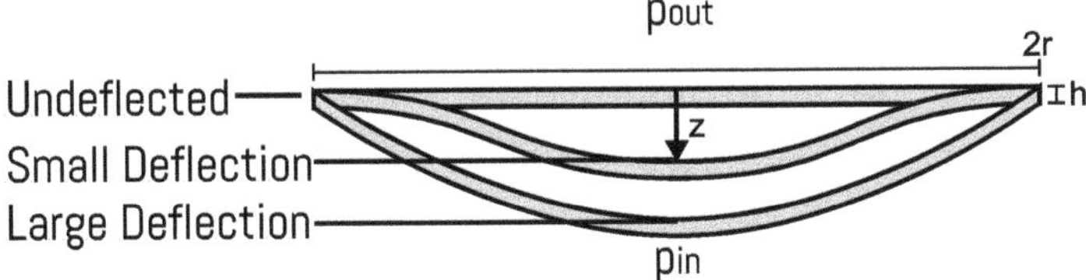

Figure 3.2: Schematic of MSD under small and large deflection, where the resistance to deformation is governed by bending and stretching respectively. r is the radius of the circular MSD, h is the thickness of the MSD and z is the center deflection of the MSD resulting from the pressure difference between p_{out} and p_{in}. The deflection is exaggerated for visibility. Small for $z \ll h$, large for $z \gg h$

The relationship between the pressure difference across a clamped, circular, flat MSD (plate for small and large deformation) and its elastic deflection is given by [38]:

$$\frac{(p_{out} - p_{in})r^4}{Eh^4} = \frac{16z}{3(1-\nu^2)h} + \frac{(7-\nu)z^3}{3(1-\nu)h^3} \tag{3.2}$$

where (see fig. 3.2):

- r is the radius of the circular MSD,
- h is the thickness of the MSD
- z is the deflection of the MSD at its center
- E is the Young's modulus of the MSD material
- ν is the Poisson's ratio of the MSD material
- Observes bending and straining

Purely elastic material behaviour is considered here. Additional considerations with respect to the viscoelastic behaviour of polymers are discussed later (see ch. 3.3).

The deflection volume ΔV_D, the volume between the undeflected and deflected state can be calculated by [38]:

$$\Delta V_D = \pi c r^2 z \tag{3.3}$$

with

$$c = \frac{C+1}{2(C+3)} \tag{3.4}$$

and

$$C = \frac{3.1|z|}{h} + \frac{3}{1+(|z|/h)^2} \tag{3.5}$$

with $c = 1/2$ for large deflection ($z >> h$) and $c = 1/3$ for small deflection ($z << h$) [38].

For small deflections, the deformation is governed by the bending of the MSD. For large deflections, stretching of the MSD becomes the limiting factor.

3.2.2 Pressure Transmission Fluid

In the context of an MSPSE, the MSD is supported by the pressure transmission fluid. The pressure difference across the MSD becomes the difference between the outer pressure and the pressure of the pressure transmission fluid, and the deflection volume is equal to the volume loss of the pressure transmission fluid under compression. To minimize the pressure difference between the outside and the inside, minimal deflection of the MSD is desired. Minimal deflection is achieved by minimal compressibility of the pressure transmission fluid. Thus, liquids are generally preferred over gases. The volume change under pressure for liquids is given by:

$$\Delta V_D = -\Delta V_{comp} = -\beta V_0 (p_{in} - p_{in}^0) \tag{3.6}$$

where:

- ΔV_{comp} is the volume change of the pressure transmission liquid,
- β is the (adiabatic) compressibility coefficient
- V_0 is the volume of the pressure transmission liquid for $p_{in} = p_{out}$
- p_{in} the pressure inside the MSPSE
- p_{in}^0 is the pressure of the pressure transmission liquid for $p_{in} = p_{out}$

For small pressures, this compressibility has a negligible effect. The assembly of the MSPSE however may leave a small air bubble trapped inside the cavity with the pressure transmission liquid. In this case the deflection volume is equal to the volume change of the trapped air bubble (fig. 3.3). Using the ideal gas law and constant temperature:

$$p_{in}^0 V_{bubble}^0 = nRT = p_{in} V_{bubble} = p_{in}(V_{bubble}^0 + \Delta V_{comp}) \tag{3.7}$$

where:

- p_{in}^0 is the pressure inside the MSPSE for $p_{in} = p_{out}$
- V_{bubble}^0 is the volume of the trapped air bubble for $p_{in} = p_{out}$
- n is the amount of substance
- R is the ideal gas constant
- T is the temperature
- p_{in} is the pressure inside the MSPSE
- V_{bubble} is the volume of the bubble
- ΔV_{comp} is the volume change of the bubble

resulting in:

$$\Delta V_D = -\Delta V_{comp} = -V_{bubble}^0 (\frac{p_{in}^0}{p_{in}} - 1) \tag{3.8}$$

When an external pressure is applied, the MSD deflects, reducing the available volume inside the capsule. This causes a compression of the air bubble and results in a pressure increase inside the capsule. This process continues until the eq. 3.3 and eq. 3.8 are fulfilled. A numerical example is given in Figure 3.4 with an applied outer pressure of 110 kPa. The blue (downwards-trending) lines show the relationship between the internal pressure and the deflection volume for different MSD diameters for the given external pressure. The red (upwards-trending) curves show the relationship between the volume change of a trapped air bubble and the internal pressure for different bubble diameters, where the diameter refers to the bubble diameter at 100 kPa. The equilibrium point for any MSD- and bubble diameter can be found at the intersection of their respective curves, where the internal pressure is matched and the bubble volume change equals the deflection volume. The difference between the applied external pressure and the equilibrium internal pressure is the pressure transmission error introduced by the encapsulation. It can be seen, that the pressure transmission error decreases with decreasing bubble diameter and increasing membrane diameter. An increase in external pressure would shift the blue (downwards-trending) curves upwards, resulting in a larger pressure transmission error, but not affect the red (upwards-trending) curves.

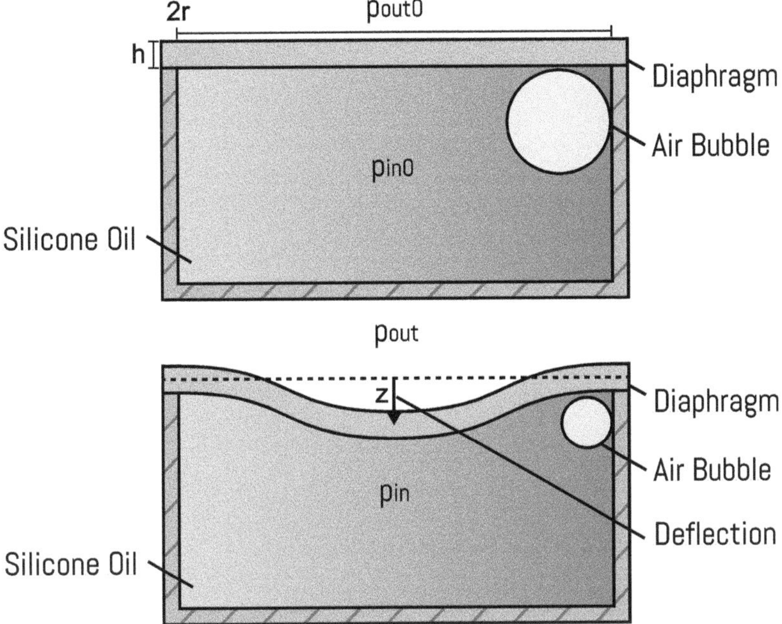

Figure 3.3: Schematic of an encapsulated air bubble with an undeflected MSD (top) and deflected MSD (bottom) as reaction to an external pressure increase. The volume change of the bubble corresponds to the deflection volume of the MSD, assuming the liquid to be incompressible.

3.2.3 Pressure Transmission Model

For an MSPSE with a trapped air bubble, assuming incompressibility of the liquid, the outer pressure can be calculated from the measured pressure by combing eq. 3.2, eq. 3.3, and eq. 3.8, resulting in:

$$p_{out} = E\left(\frac{16V^0_{bubble}(1-\frac{p^0_{in}}{p_{in}})h^3}{3(\pi c)(1-\nu^2)r^6} + \frac{(7-\nu){V^0_{bubble}}^3(1-\frac{p^0_{in}}{p_{in}})^3 h}{3(\pi c)^3(1-\nu)r^{10}}\right) + p_{in} \quad (3.9)$$

The large exponents of the MSD radius r, but also of the bubble diameter ${V^0_{bubble}}^3 = (\frac{\pi d^3}{6})^3$ are main contribution factors (fig. 3.5), whereas the thickness of the MSD only has a small impact on the pressure transmission.

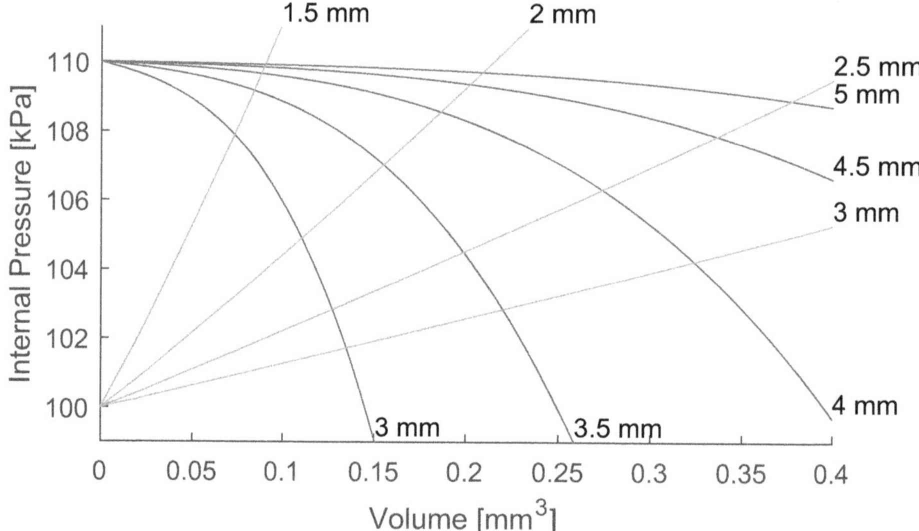

Figure 3.4: Numeric example of MSD deflection and bubble compression. The blue (downward-trending) curves show the inner pressure (p_{in}) for a given deflection volume for MSDs of different sizes, with an outer pressure (p_{out}) of 110 kPa. The red (upwards-trending) curves show the inner pressure (p_{in}) for a given volume change (compression) of the encapsulated bubble. The pressure error can be found at the intersection of any red (upwards-trending) and blue (downward-trending) curve, for different MSD and bubble diameters.

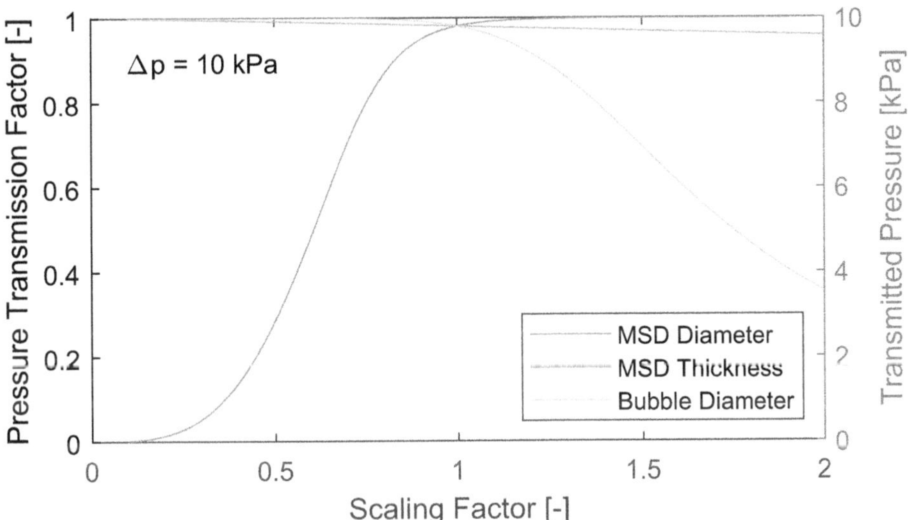

Figure 3.5: Numeric example of the influence of individual scaling of the design parameters MSD diameter and thickness, and bubble diameter for an outer pressure increase of 10 kPa. Rapid pressure transmission decay can be observed for shrinking MSDs and growing bubbles. The MSD thickness has less of an impact. Initial values: MSD diameter = 5 mm, MSD thickness = 20 μm, bubble diameter = 2 mm

3.3 Temperature Cross Sensitivity

Temperature cross sensitivity (TCS) describes changes of measured pressure induced by changes of the temperature of the capsule without change of the external pressure. This sensitivity originates from the mismatch of coefficients of thermal expansion (CTE) of the different materials used. Linear CTE of materials used for the MSPSE:

- MSD (Parylene C): $\alpha_L \approx 3.5 * 10^{-5}/K$
- Pressure transmission fluid (Si-Oil): $\alpha_L \approx 3.3 * 10^{-4}/K$
- Housing (Titanium): $\alpha_L \approx 8.6 * 10^{-6}/K$

note: isotropic material expansion is assumed, $\alpha_V = 3\alpha_L$.

The significantly larger CTE of the enclosed pressure transmission liquid causes a pressure increase inside the capsule which to some extent is dampened by the MSD.

The change in volume of a liquid:

$$\Delta V_L = \alpha_V V_{L0} \Delta T \tag{3.10}$$

This change of volume is compensated by the deflection of the MSD (eq. 3.2 and eq. 3.3).

$$(p_{Temp} - p_0) = \left(\frac{16(\Delta V_D)}{3(1-\nu^2)(\pi c r^2) h} + \frac{(7-\nu)(\Delta V_D)^3}{3(1-\nu)(\pi c r^2)^3 h^3} \right) \frac{E h^4}{r^4} \tag{3.11}$$

and volume change of the bubble,

$$\frac{p(V^0_{bubble} + \Delta V^0_{bubble})}{p_0 V^0_{bubble}} = \frac{T_0 + \Delta T}{T_0} \tag{3.12}$$

- T_0 is the temperature, where $p_{in} = p_{out}$
- V^0_{bubble} is the volume of the trapped air bubble at T_0

- V_{L0} is the volume of the transmission liquid at T_0

fulfilling over all:

$$\Delta V_D = \Delta V_{bubble} + \Delta V_L \tag{3.13}$$

$$\Delta V_D = \frac{(T_0 + \Delta T)(p_0 V^0_{bubble})}{p_{in} T_0} - V^0_{bubble} + \alpha_V V_{L0} \Delta T \tag{3.14}$$

Figure 3.6 shows a typical TCS curve. The air content is increasing the TCS, however, even a high air fraction of 10 % in the cavity volume still has a small impact on the overall TCS.

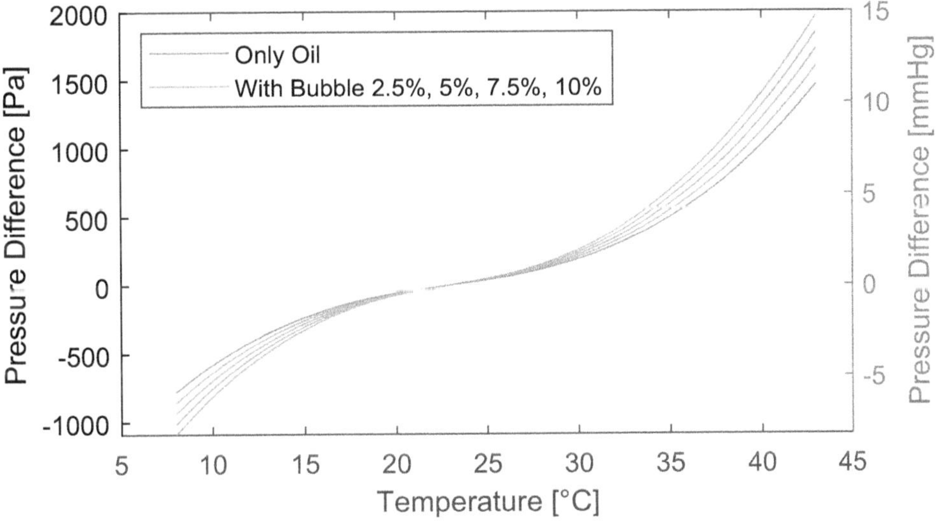

Figure 3.6: Numeric example of the influence of a trapped air bubble on the temperature cross sensitivity for different air content percentages of the capsule cavity volume. In an MSPSE with MSD diameter = 5 mm, MSD thickness = 20 μm, cavity volume = 20.9 μL. The pressure across the MSD is set to be zero at 23°. Result of 3.11 and eq. 3.14.

In figure 3.7 the effect of scaling of individual components on the TCS can be seen. The characteristic length[1] of the cavity and the MSD Diameter dominate, while both MSD thickness and air to liquid ratio have rather small

[1] The term characteristic length refers to any choosable length of the cavity and indicates that all other dimensions are scaled proportionally to the characteristic length. As such its scaling is proportional to $\sqrt[3]{Volume}$

effects on the TCS for the given initial parameter set. This means that a low TCS can be achieved by combining a large MSD with a small cavity and explains why a typical liquid filled MSPSE is designed like figure 3.1 to maximize the MSD area and minimize the liquid volume and not like the simplified figure 3.3.

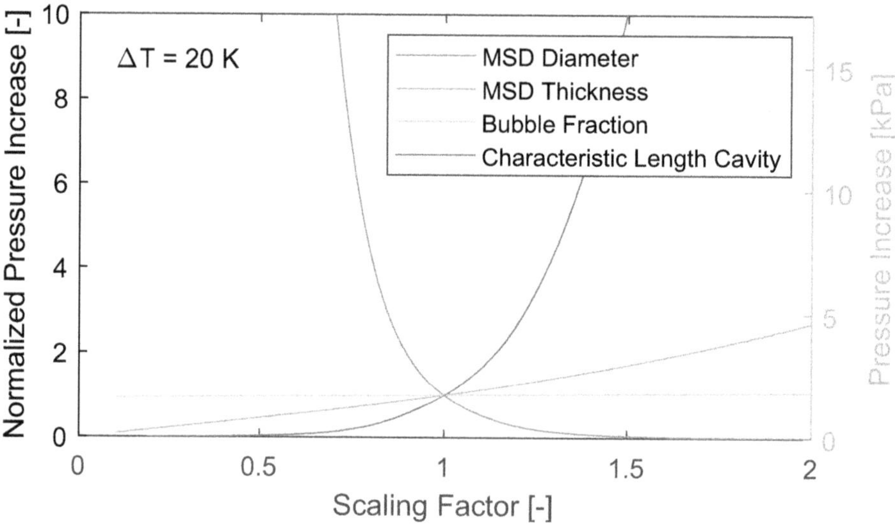

Figure 3.7: Numeric example of the influence of individual scaling of the design parameters MSD diameter and thickness, characteristic length of the cavity and the bubble fraction of the cavity volume for a temperature increase of 20 K. The MSD diameter and cavity size (1D) dominate the TCS, while the bubble fraction and MSD thickness have a negligible and small influence respectively. Initial values: MSD diameter = 5 mm, MSD thickness = 20 μm, bubble fraction = 2.5 %, characteristic length cavity = $\sqrt[3]{21\mu L}$

3.4 Drift

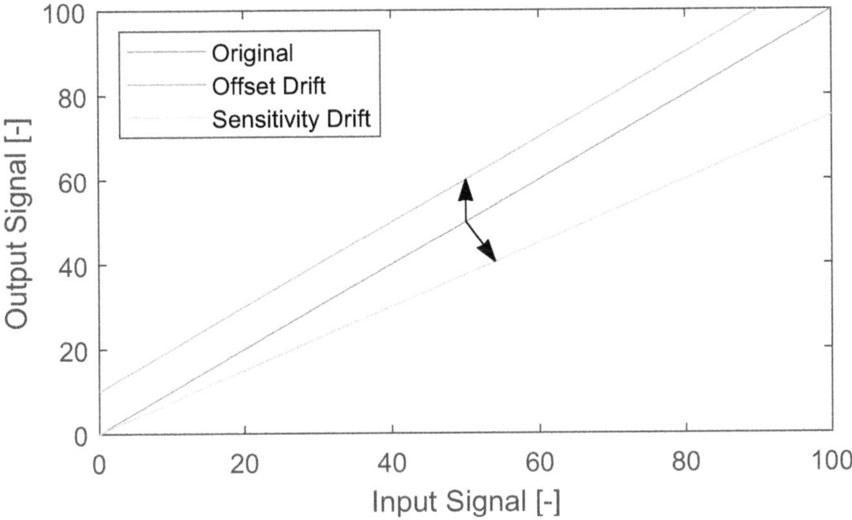

Figure 3.8: Schematic example of offset and sensitivity drift.

Drift describes a slow change of the system over time and is often split into offset-drift and sensitivity-drift as displayed in figure 3.8. Reviewing all previously shown equations, the following causes for drift can be anticipated:

- Change of material properties E, ν, α_L (e.g.: ageing, corrosion, swelling)
- Change of MSD thickness h (e.g.: swelling)
- Loss/gain of pressure transmission fluid in the capsule V_L (e.g.: leakage, diffusion into capsule)
- Viscoelastic behaviour of the polymer MSD

3.5 Viscoelasticity

Viscoelasticity is a material property describing a time dependent stress/strain relation and expresses itself in two ways: Straining of the material results in an immediate elastic stress response which slowly decays to some extent over time (fig. 3.10, fig. 3.11). Or, stressing of the material results in an elastic strain response which continues to some extent over time.

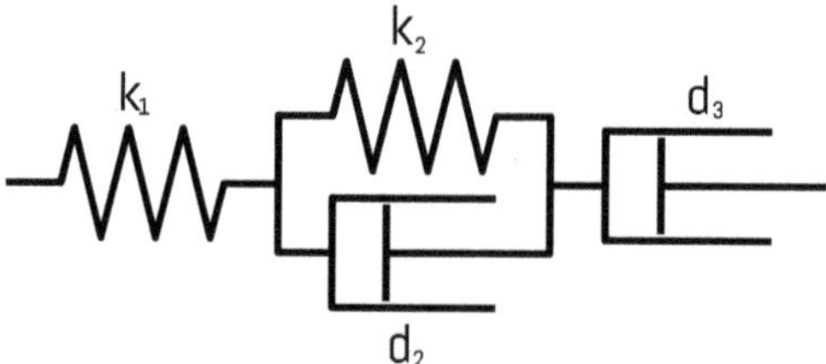

Figure 3.9: Schematic representation of the Burgers model, with the purely elastic component on the left k_1, the viscoelastic component in the center $k_2 \& d_2$ and a purely viscous component d_3 at the end.

Mathematically, viscoelasticity can be expressed as a combination of springs and dashpots (dampener). The Burgers model (fig. 3.9), a combination of the Maxwell and Kelvin-Voigt model has been found to represent the viscoelastic properties of Parylene well [39]. The Burgers model in its basic form consists of a series of a spring, a parallel spring/dashpot element and a dashpot (fig. 3.9). The spring reflecting the purely elastic behaviour, the parallel spring/dashpot element reflecting the viscoelastic behaviour and the dashpot reflecting viscous behaviour or creep. In this model, the strain of a material is represented as total elongation of all elements of the model chain, while stress corresponds to the force exerted by the spring element.

Figure 3.10 shows a simulated example of a viscoelastic material as modelled by the Burgers model. In this example, strain is applied and stress is observed. The model shows the decay of stress after reaching a maximum as the strain is applied. In this simulation the spring constants of the pure spring k_1 and the combined spring/dashpot element k_2 have been set to 1. Due to the non-instantaneous strain application, the stress never reaches 1, as would be expected for a pure spring with k = 1, since the spring/dashpot element already had time to elongate during the straining process. The elongation of the pure spring and combined spring/dashpot elements is shown in the lower part of the figure. As elongation is the set parameter, the two elements are required to have a combined total elongation of 1. The time dependence introduced by the combined spring/dashpot element can be observed, as it elongates only slowly due to force exerted onto the chain by the pure spring component under its initial peak elongation. While for instantaneous elongation, the combined spring/dashpot element acts as a rigid element and does not elongate, for infinite time it acts as a pure spring. In the lower part of figure 3.10, this can be observed as the two elements reach equal length and therefore also equal force over the course of time (time mark: 6). When

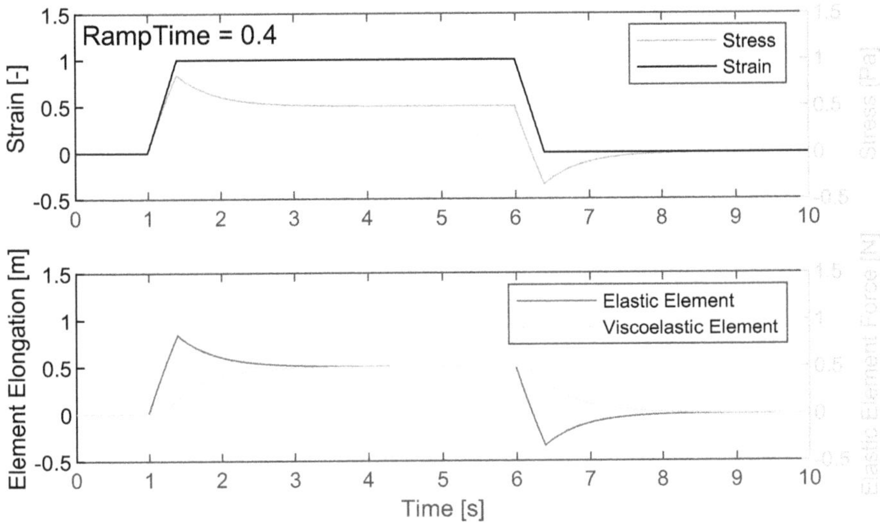

Figure 3.10: Numeric example of the Burgers model. Top: Example of a viscoelastic material's reaction to strain. After expanding (i.e. straining) the material to a fixed length, the initially high stress decays to a certain level over time. Upon reversion of the expansion, negative stress is experienced by the material, which decays until the initial state is re-established. Bottom: Length readjustment over time of the elastic and viscoelastic component in the model until an equilibrium (equal force) is reached. Upon reversion of the expansion, both components revert slowly to their initial size.

the strain of the modelled material is returned to its initial state, the reverse process occurs. The combined spring/dashpot element at first opposes the deformation and remains in its elongated state and only returns to its initial state over time. The stress/strain curve for the simulated material for different ramping times can be seen in figure 3.11. It is visible that for flatter strain ramps, the stress significantly decays during the ramping.

3.5.1 Implications for this Project

The MSPSE inherits the viscoelastic properties of the MSD material. This can be interpreted as follows: The temperature induced expansion of the transmission fluid strains the MSD and is thus proportional to the elongation in the model chain. The stress which the MSD experiences is reverted back to the pressure transmission fluid as pressure, which can be interpreted as the force in the model. This implies that a temperature increase results in

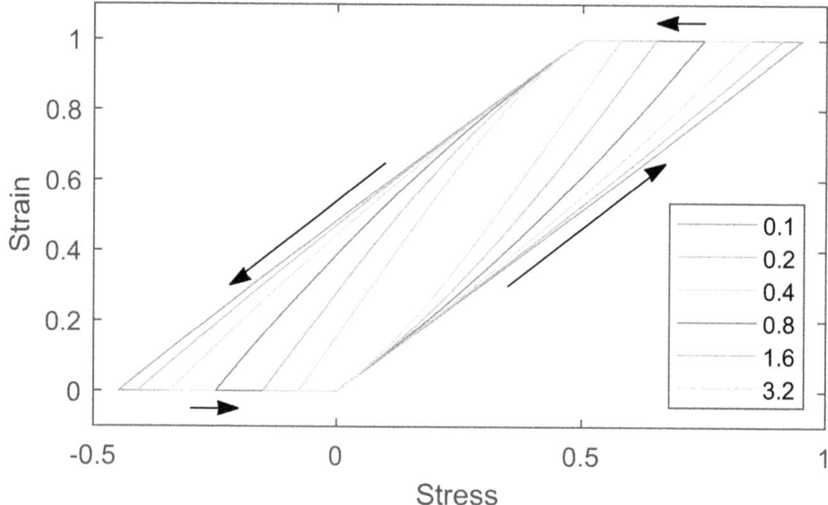

Figure 3.11: Numeric example of the Burgers model. Stress-strain loop for a viscoelastic material and various ramp times (see fig. 3.10). In this example, the strain is controlled and the stress is the result of the applied strain. Unlike a purely elastic material, the time spent at each expansion point shifts the stress-strain curve.

a pressure increase, which decays over time. This behaviour will be referred to as temperature induced (offset) drift.

While high pressure transmission and low temperature cross sensitivity are fundamentally desirable, the time dependent nature of viscoelasticity poses a more complex challenge for error correction. In a purely elastic system, both pressure transmission and temperature cross sensitivity can easily be corrected by either mathematical function or interpolated lookup-tables. In a viscoelastic system however, not only the momentary temperature needs to be known, but also the state of the system (i.e. the elongation of each used component of the Burgers Model), which is the result of the history of applied pressures and temperatures it experienced.

In the context of MSPSE the error decays for both pressure transmission and temperature cross sensitivity. Temperature cross sensitivity is strain driven as described above.

Pressure transmission, while stress driven, also results in a decay of the pressure transmission error over time. Here the applied stress (resulting from the pressure difference across the MSD) causes a viscoelastic straining of the MSD, which increases the deflection volume over time and thus, the pressure transmission, but reduce the pressure transmission error by moving the system closer towards the true value (fig. 3.4, red (upward-trending) line towards larger volume).

In general, measuring a variable proportional to the decaying side of a viscoelastic couple like stress/strain or force/length will result in a decrease of error, while measuring the variable proportional to the other will result in an increasing error. The opposite is true if the error is the complement of the measured variable, such as is the case for the pressure transmission error.

For MSPSEs this means that if the maximal pressure transmission error and temperature induced pressure offset can be designed to be within the error tolerance, the error will not exceed the boundaries due to viscoelasticity independent of the time of observation.

3.6 Analysis of Previous Demonstrator Device

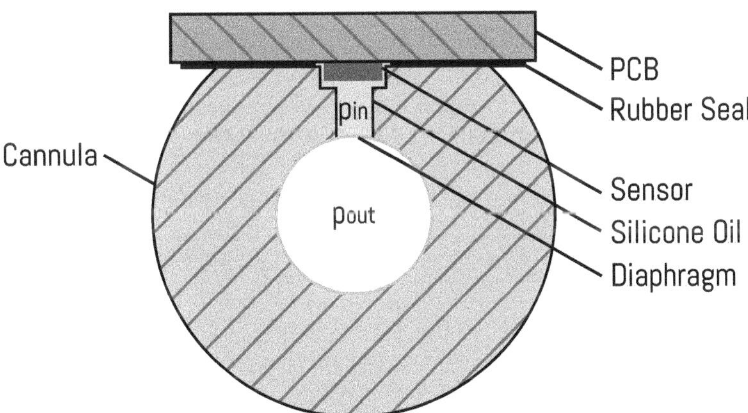

Figure 3.12: Schematic cross-section through the demonstrator device. The PCB at the top is pressed against the cannula, sandwitching a rubber seal. The MSD diameter is fixed to the lower diameter of the capsule cavity. (Device as described in [30])

In previous work, Staufert et. al [30] developed a MSD-in-coating concept, which enabled the integration of a commercial pressure sensor into a cannula, while maintaining a seamless blood-contacting interface (fig 3.12). There, a small area of the Parylene-C coating was used to transmit pressure. This was achieved by filling the pressure transmission channel with a sacrificial material before coating (fig. 3.14). Maintaining a smooth inner wall of the cannula is expected to reduce turbulences and therefore negative interactions with blood. Furthermore the cavity of the device was designed with the goal of eliminating trapping of air bubbles during the filling process to maximize pressure transmission. This was achieved by combining electrical feedthrough and backside sealing into the same physical element, thereby reducing the complexity of the cavity.

3.6.1 Challenges

Temperature cross sensitivity was not considered for the demonstrator. Figure 3.13 shows the predicted purely elastic TCS. The used fabrication process does not allow for independent sizing of the pressure transmission channel diameter and MSD size, which is required to reduce the TCS.

The process used to prepare the cannulas for Parylene coating by plugging the pressure transmission channel to create a smooth inner surface inside the cannula was found to suffer from few failure modes as described by Staufert [40]. The process consisted of four steps: First, a cylindrical core with higher CTE than the cannula material was placed inside the cannula at room temperature. Second, cannula and core were heated above the melting temperature of the sacrificial plugging material (wax). This caused the core to extend and press against the inner wall of the cannula, sealing the pressure transmission channel off. The molten wax was then pored into the pressure transmission channel. Third, the assembly was slowly cooled down to allow the wax to solidify to a plug and shrink the core back to its original size and become removable. Finally the core was removed, leaving the solidified sacrificial wax plug in place, creating a seamless inner surface of the cannula, which could then be used to deposit Parylene. Four failure modes were observed with this process and are schematically depicted in figure 3.15: Leakage of the sacrificial material into small gaps between the core and the cannula (fig. 3.15 a), non-ideal replication of the core surface (fig. 3.15 b), enclosed bubbles at the interface between wax and core resulting in large cavities in the wax plug's surface (fig. 3.15 c), cracking of the plug and/or delamination of the plug from the pressure transmission channel (fig. 3.15 d) was observed as described in [40]. When multiple channels in a single device need to be plugged synchronously, the chance of all of them succeeding is drastically reduced, reducing the per-device yield.

Finally, the sealing process (see fig. 3.14) appears to be very sensitive. Little "over tightening" past the point of full sealing drastically increases the pressure inside the cavity (fig. 3.16). Furthermore, the point of full sealing depends on the pressure difference accross the seal (fig. 3.12), meaning that overtightening is required during assembly to compensate for the expected higher pressures in the pressure transmission liquid during operation. During the assembly process, as the point of full sealing is approached, the overpressure decay due to leakage of excess pressure transmission liquid becomes infinitely slow, rendering this process in need of further improvement.

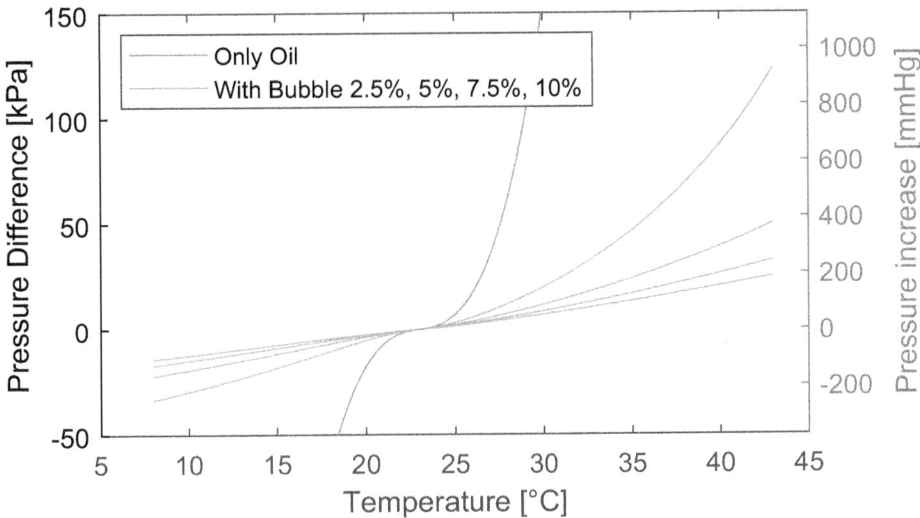

Figure 3.13: Calculated purely elastic temperature cross sensitivity of the demonstrator device for pure oil and multiple trapped air fractions.

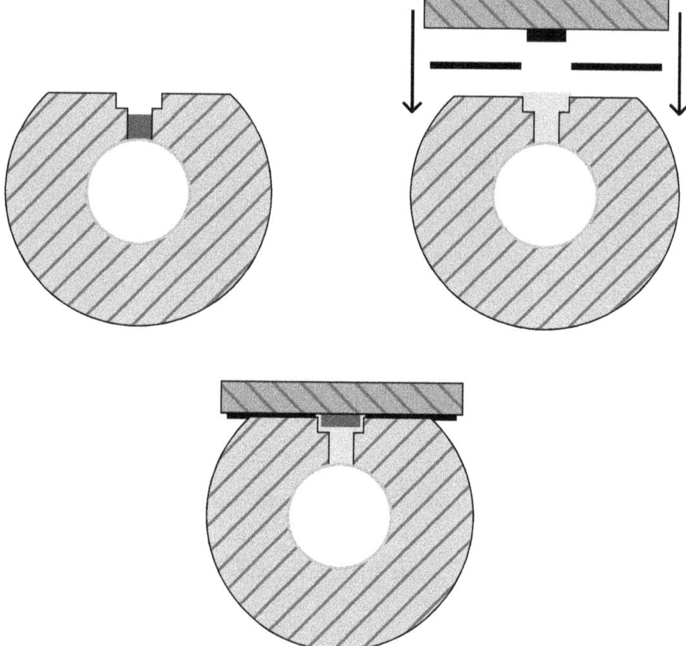

Figure 3.14: Schematic of the assembly processes of the demonstrator device. Top-left: Wax plug inside the pressure transmission channel (purple) for the Parylene layer coating. Top right: sealing process after oil-fill. Bottom: assembled and sealed device. (Assembly as performed for [30], to the best of the authors knowledge)

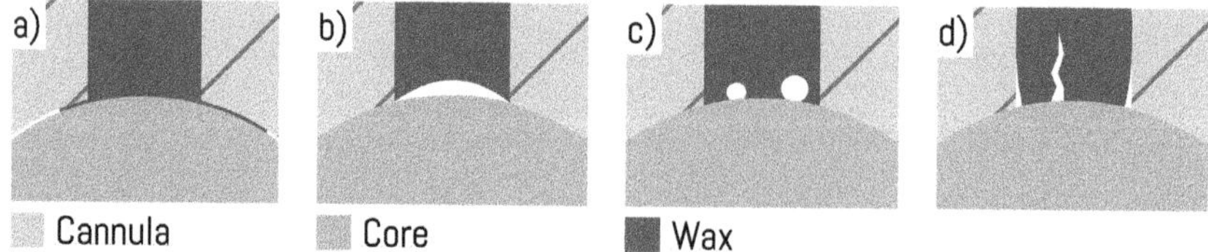

Figure 3.15: Schematic of the observed failure modes of the wax plug method. a) Leakage of wax onto the inner surface of the cannula. b) Solidification shrinkage resulting in concave wax plug surface. c) Trapped air bubbles, resulting in cavities at the core surface. d) Cracking of the plug or delamination from the pressure transmission channel, as a result of thermal and solidification shrinkage. Adapted from [40].

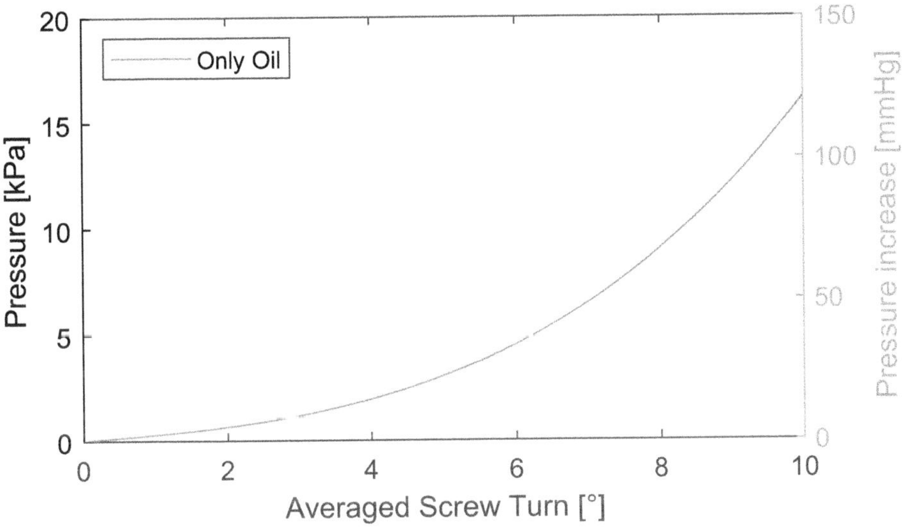

Figure 3.16: Calculated pressure increase during the sealing process for screwing angles after sealing is achieved due to rubber seal compression. Assuming each screw turn is equally spread across each of the 4 screws (1/4).

3.7 MSD Design for Implants

The size of the MSD has a significant impact on the characteristics of the MSPSE such as pressure transmission and TCS. Additionally to size constraints by the implantable testing platform's main body, the curvature of the MSD needs to be considered.

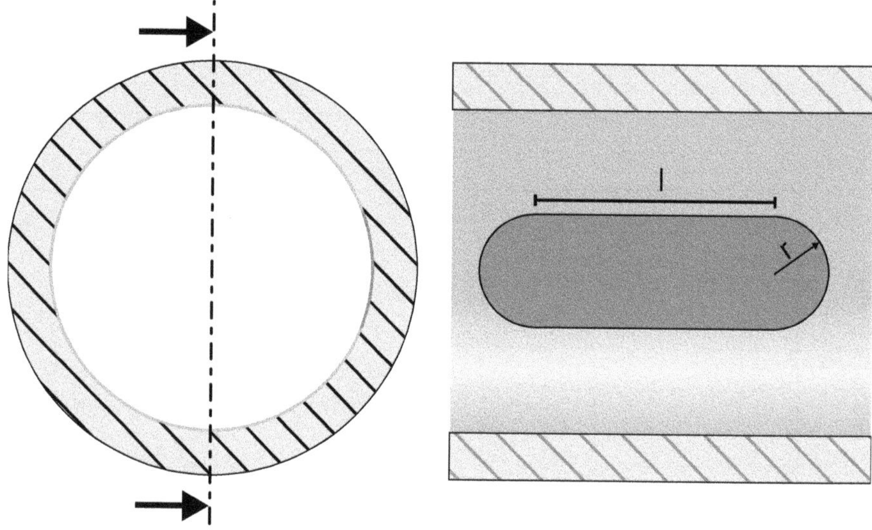

Figure 3.17: Schematic of a pill shaped MSD placed in the inside of a pipe. Left: side view showing the curvature of the MSD. Right: Top view, showing the pill-shape of the MSD. l is the length of the rectangular middle section, r is is the radius of the circular end parts of the MSD.

The target pressure acquisition point for VAD control is on the inner wall of the cylindrical or conical inflow cannula. Therefore any MSD integrated in the coating of such an inflow cannula would inherit its curvature (see fig. 3.17). To mimic this curvature, the implantable testing platform (see ch. 4.2) discussed in this work was designed in the form of a pipe, on which's inner wall $r_i = 5\ mm$, the pressure was to be measured. For flat MSDs a larger MSD is beneficial both for a high pressure transmission (ch. 3.2) as well as for a low temperature cross sensitivity (ch. 3.3). For curved MSDs however, the incremental benefit can be severely reduced depending on the radius of the cylinder [40]. To reduce the influence of the curvature the radial dimension was limited to 3.76 mm, while elongating the MSD along the axis of the cylinder of the implantable testing platform, resulting in a pill shaped MSD with a total length of 11.76 mm.[2] The deflection volume was calculated as the sum of the deflection volume of the circular MSD and a rectangular MSD part, placed in-between and given the same deflection[3] as the cross-section of the circular MSD:

$$\Delta V_D = \pi c r^2 z + 2lczr \tag{3.15}$$

Replacing ΔV_D in eq. 3.14 and solving for p_{in} gives;

$$p_{in} = \frac{(T_0 + \Delta T) p_0 V^0_{bubble}}{T_0 (cz\pi r^2 + 2lczr + V^0_{bubble} - \alpha_V V_{L0} \Delta T)} \tag{3.16}$$

An estimate for the bubble size V^0_{bubble} was found via ideal gas law, by assuming, that the trapped air mass is equal to the air mass filling the cavity at the lowest pressure during the oil-fill process (see fig. 5.24), i.e.:

$$V^0_{bubble} = \frac{p_{vac} V_{tot}}{p_{ambient}} \tag{3.17}$$

The free parameters r and l were chosen to be 1.88 mm and 8 mm to keep a TCS of 268 Pa (2 mmHg) within the temperature operating window (see fig. 3.18). The pressure transmission is shown in figure 3.19 and is calculated to be 74 Pa (0.6 mmHg) for the pressure operating window.

Table 3.1 lists the material properties, operating range and design parameters used for the implantable testing platform. The p_{vac} refers to the lowest achievable vacuum pressure during the oil-filling step. p_{op} and T_{op} refer to the operating range of the MSPSE after implantation. V_{tot}, the cavity volume of the MSPSE was given by other construction constraints, such as the diameter of the oil-fill and pressure transmission channel. The thickness of 20 μm was chosen for robustness of the MSD, leaving only the shape of the MSD to be defined.

[2] The exact values were chosen to maintain a TCS of less than ± 1 mmHg from 35°C to 45°C, based on the model described here, while minimizing the effect of curvature [40] (see ch. 3.7.1). The length was limited by the space available in the axial direction of the implant.

[3] Conservative assumption: the deflection profile is likely larger for a given pressure, therefore accepting a larger volume or resulting in a lower pressure increase for the same volume change.

Table 3.1: Material properties, operating range and design parameters used in this work.

Property	Value	Description
E	$2.76\ GPa$	**Young's Modulus, from: [41]**
ν	0.4	**Poisson's Ratio**
$\alpha_{v,oil}$	$10 * 10^{-4} 1/K$	**Vol. CTE of Si-Oil**
p_{vac}	$2\ kPa$	**Residual vacuum pressure**
p_{op}	$-2.7\ kPa\ to\ 26.7\ kPa$	**Relative pressure range**
T_{op}	$35°C\ to\ 42°C$	**Operating temperature range**
V_{tot}	$20.9\ mm^3$	**Capsule cavity volume**
h	$20\ \mu m$	**MSD thickness**
r	$1.88\ mm$	**Pill radius**
l	$8\ mm$	**Pill length**

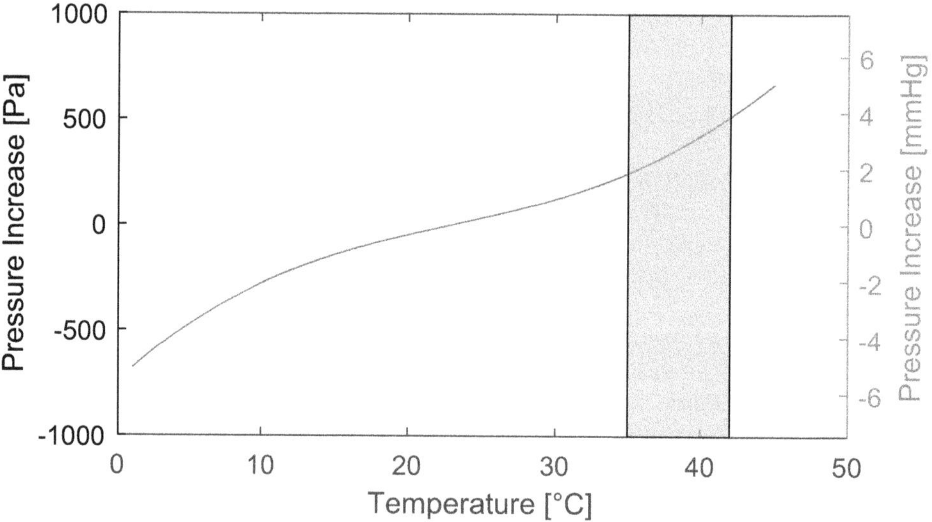

Figure 3.18: Calculated temperature cross sensitivity for a flat pill shaped MSD with r = 1.88 mm, l = 8 mm, h = 20 µm. The blue, shaded area marks the operation temperature range.

3.7.1 Model vs. Reality

The fabricated MSD deviates from the model in three points: First, only the CTE of the pressure transmission fluid was included. The CTE of the MSD and titanium housing were neglected. Second, the curvature of the MSD was

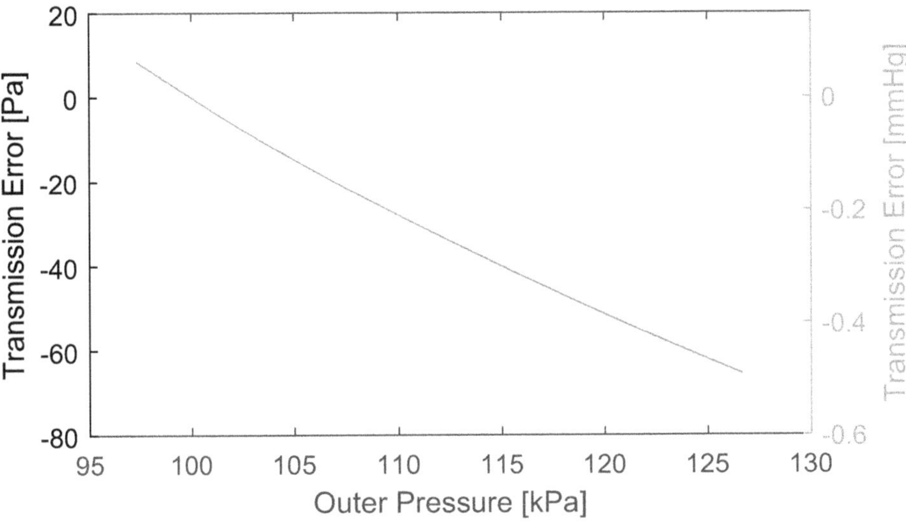

Figure 3.19: Calculated pressure transmission error for a flat pill shaped MSD with r = 1.88 mm, l = 8 mm, h = 20 µm.

neglected. Third, the deflection profile and centre deflection was assumed to be the same for the pill-shaped MSD as it would be for a circular MSD.

Neglecting the CTE of the Parylene MSD and titanium housing, in the case of a flat MSD, was expected to result in an overestimation of the TCS. The expansion of the titanium housing compensates the expansion of the pressure transmission fluid to some extent. Due to the large difference in CTE (Ti: ca. 26E-6 1/K (volumetric) and Si-Oil 10E-4 1/K (volumetric)) this effect is expected to remain neglectable. The CTE of Parylene lies in-between (ca. 10.5E-5 1/K (volumetric) [42]), which makes it more relevant for two reasons. First, the CTE of Parylene is closer to that of Si-Oil, second it is larger than that of the titanium housing and the MSD is fixed to the housing in its perimeter. The later reason means that with increasing temperature, the MSD expands more than the housing, becomes large than its perimeter fixture and naturally supports the creation of a deflection volume. This effect is expected to be strongest around zero deflection. For a flat MSD, these effects are therefore all expected to result in a lower TCS than predicted. In the case of a curved MSD it is possible that the expansion of the Parylene creates an increased TCS until partial buckling is initiated.

The effect of curvature of an MSD placed inside a pipe was simulated by Staufert [40] and predicted to depend on the ratio between width of the MSD in radial direction of the pipe and the pipe's diameter. The chosen combination of width and pipe diameter place this MSD in an area where a width increase would offer little benefit, which in turn means a larger pipe diameter would offer a lower TCS. Despite the expected curvature effect, a larger width was still expected to result in a lower overall TCS.

The shape of the deflected pill shaped MSD is expected to slightly deviate from the model. The rectangular middle section is expected to have a higher centre deflection than a circular MSD for the same load. In the combined case, a transition towards the semi-circular ends is expected. However, overall the model is expected to underrepresent the deflection volume and overestimate the TCS.

4 Approach of the Thesis

A colored version of this chapter is available at: https://doi.org/10.3929/ethz-b-000702759

4.1 Goals

The main goal of this project was to produce a cylindrical implantable testing platform based on the MSD-in-coating concept [30]. The implantable testing platform, an assembly of multiple so called sensor capsules, for measuring blood pressure had to be capable of in-vivo operation over a period of 3 months and containing as many MSPSEs as possible to maximize the data per animal. Additionally, the device was required to maintain a maximum compensated total error of ± 3 mmHg (accuracy) over this period without recalibration.

In order to reduce the impact of viscoelasticity, the capsules were to be designed such that temperature fluctuations in the body (35°C to 42°C) would not cause the error to exceed the limits even without correction.

Furthermore, an assembly pressure minimizing solution for the sealing after filling had to be found. Minimal preload on the MSD should also result in minimal viscoelastic post-assembly drift and reduce the risk of damage to the MSD.

Additionally, the yield of the MSD production step had to be improved to enable the production of multi-capsule devices.

4.2 Implantable Testing Platform

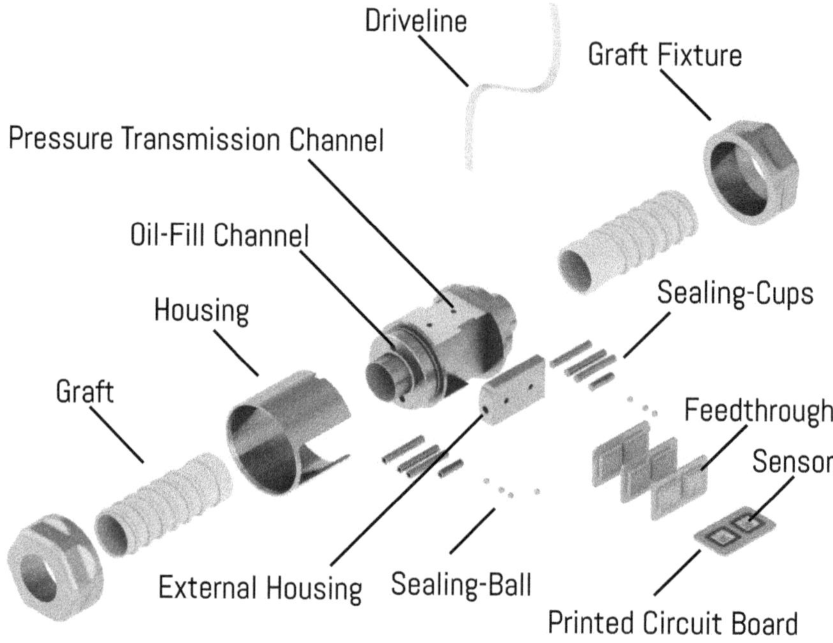

Figure 4.1: Exploded view of the implantable testing platform for multiple MSPSE.

The implantable testing platform (fig. 4.1) consists of a pipe like body through which blood can flow. The blood contacting inner side is coated with Parylene in which six MSDs are embedded. Each MSD covers its own pressure transmission channel through the wall of the body. An electrical feedthrough package containing a sensor was fixed on the other side of each pressure transmission channel. Sealing of the oil-fill channel, which was placed in the wall of the main body in parallel to the pipe direction, was achieved by a ball-cup sealing. Each end of the pipe body was shaped into a thin walled connector over which a graft could be pulled and fixed with the graft fixtures. A cross-section through one of the sensor encapsulations formed by the body, electrical feedthrough, MSD, and backside sealing can be seen in figure 4.2. The MSD is embedded in the Parylene coating at the bottom of the pressure transmission channel and the electrical feedthrough at the top. The oil-fill and pressure transmission channel's centre axes are offset and the channel only overlaps in a small area to allow pressure transmission after placing the sealing cups in the oil-fill channel. Two equivalent assemblies with the MSD facing outwards of the device were embedded in the external sensor housing to measure the ambient pressure. This work focuses on the six inward facing MSPSEs capable of measuring blood pressure.

An electrical schematic of the sensor readout electronics can be found in figure 4.3. The multiplexor and sensors are controlled by an MSP 430 microcontroller by I2C interface. The acquired measurement data is passed to a PC by serial interface. The multiplexor is required, as the sensors can only have two distinct I2C addresses. The readout cycle consists of opening the multiplexor channel, reading the stored measurement and starting a new measurement on both connected sensors, then closing the channel and proceeding to the next channel. The sensors can then acquire a new measurement while the microcontroller moves through the other multiplexor channels. At the end of every cycle the acquired data is sent to the PC.

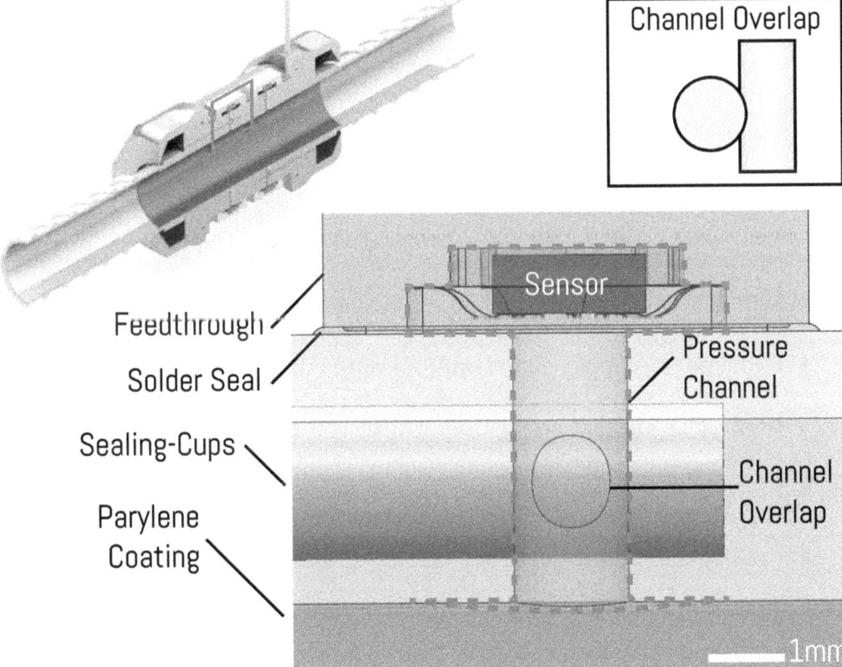

Figure 4.2: Cross-section view through one of the MSPSE. The dashed red line represents the boundaries of the capsule in which the oil is enclosed. The inset shows the relative offset of the oil-fill channel to the pressure transmission channel.

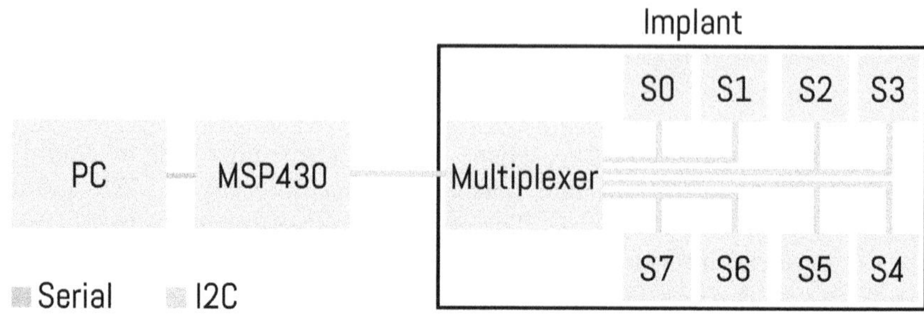

Figure 4.3: Layout of the sensor readout electronics system. The sensors and a multiplexer is placed inside the implant. Sensors 0-5 are enclosed in inward facing MSPSEs and Sensors 6 and 7 in outward facing MSPSEs. The multiplexer is connected to a microcontroller via the drive line and the microcontroller is connected to a laptop. Communication between the microcontroller and the laptop uses a serial interface and the microcontroller uses I2C with the multiplexer and sensors.

4.3 MSD

The target properties for the MSD were defined as:

- Improved MSD adhesion
- Decoupling of MSD shape and pressure transmission channel diameter
- High yield parallel and/or repeatable serial process MSD fabrication
- High pressure transmission
- Leak free MSD

A major challenge to the application of Parylene as coating for implants is the poor long term adhesion of Parylene to many common implant materials, such as titanium. Staufert et al. developed a solution based on mechanical interlocking of titanium-oxide nanostructures with Parylene [40]. The nanostructure anchoring was shown to fully eliminate the delamination of Parylene on titanium, to the point of destruction of the Parylene layer [40]. This solution was used in this work to ensure that the MSD retains its shape over the duration of the implantation.

TCS is most significantly governed by the ratio of pressure transmission fluid volume over MSD area (see fig. 3.7).

In the demonstrator device [30] the pressure transmission channel and MSD diameter were locked to be the same. In order to reduce the TCS, these two diameters had to be decoupled. Two approaches compatible with nanostructure anchoring were explored for this purpose, both with the intent to create a freely designable MSD area within the Parylene coating. The first approach was to cover and block the nanostructures from interlocking with the Parylene at defined areas during coating. The second approach was to locally remove the nanostructures and create an area of controlled delamination to form the MSD (ch. 5.1).

Alternatives to the previously used [30] process to plug the pressure transmission channel before Parylene coating were explored. A plug free approach and multiple alternatives of forming the plug were explored based on thermal, chemical and dehydration based solid-liquid transition, as well as a transition free powder compression based approach (ch. 5.2).

As for all other parts leakage free operation is mandatory for the MSD. This is especially important for the MSD due to its contact to blood. Helium leakage tests for the MSD process were applied [43].

4.4 Pressure Transmission Fluid

The target property for the enclosed pressure transmission fluid was defined as:

- low gas content

Pressure transmission is most significantly governed by the ratio of gaseous content in the cavity over MSD area (see fig. 3.5). The demonstrator device [30] solved this by designing the cavity in a fashion that allowed complete evacuation during the oil filling process. In this work, complete evaquability was sacrificed for separability of backside sealing and electrical feedthrough and overall form factor of the device. High pressure transmission was pursued by aiming at maintaining a sufficiently low ratio of gaseous content in the cavity over MSD area (fig. 3.5).

4.5 Electrical Feedthrough

The target properties for the electrical feedthrough were defined as:

- sufficient electrical channels
- hermetic sealing
- rigid

In this work another sensor to the one used in the demonstrator of Staufert et al. [30] was used due to its smaller form factor. This sensor (LPS 22 Fam, STMicroelectronics) is I2C capable, requiring four electric interconnects.

Hermetic sealing of all components is crucial for the long-term drift-free operation of MSPSE. Even minuscule leakage rates and the resulting loss of pressure transmission fluid can cause significant offset-drift over time. Parylene compatible solder-sealing and helium leakage tests for the electrical feedthrough process were applied [44].

As for every component of the capsule that is not in contact with the medium whose pressure is to be measured, high rigidity is important as any deflection would work against the MSD's deflection, reducing the pressure transmission or resulting in offset-drift. Here, ceramics and a solder-based approach was used for this purpose (ch. 5.3).

4.6 Backside Sealing

The target properties for the backside sealing were defined as:

- minimal assembly pressure increase
- hermetic sealing
- rigid

Low assembly pressure increase is especially important in the context of viscoelasticity where the pressure increase would decay over time, potentially resulting in significant drift. Here a ball-cup-sealing was used (ch. 5.4).

For hermetic sealing and rigidity, the same rational applies as described in section 4.5. Helium-leak testing of this component was also used to verify its reliability [45].

5 Individual Components

This chapter discusses the fabrication of the individual components of the sensor encapsulation and their properties as functional groups. Figure 5.1 gives an overview over the interlaced MSPSE fabrication process flow.

A colored version of this chapter is available at: https://doi.org/10.3929/ethz-b-000702759

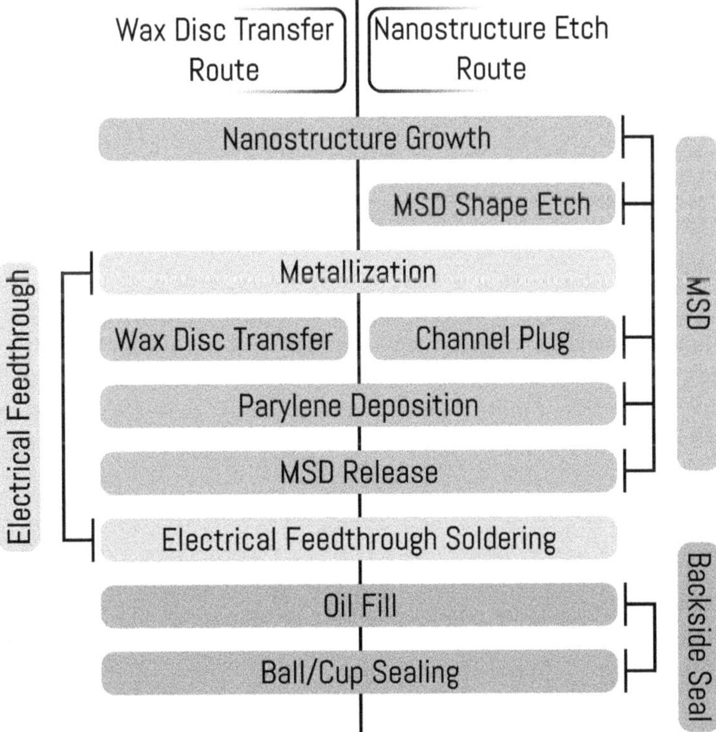

Figure 5.1: Overview of the MSPSE production workflow. Left: Wax disc route, right: Nanostructure etching route.

5.1 MSD

5.1.1 MSD Shape

To enable MSD shaping and sizing independently of the pressure transmission channel two approaches were explored (fig. 5.2). The first, here referred to as wax disc transfer route, aims at preventing the mechanical interlocking of Parylene and titanium nanostructures in a defined area during the deposition process by means of a sacrificial layer. The sacrificial layer was preshaped on a transfer sheet and placed above the pressure transmission channel before coating. Release of the MSD after coating occurred by dissolution of the sacrificial material. The second approach, here referred to as nanostructure etch route, is based on the low intrinsic adhesion of Parylene on unstructured titanium. Nanostructures in a specified area around the pressure transmission channel were etched away using photolithography based techniques before Parylene coating. Release of the MSD in the etched area was achieved by application of air pressure via the pressure transmission channel.

5.1.2 Materials & Methods

For all MSDs, nanostructures were first grown on titanium samples as described in [40]. Four types of samples were used: cubes (6 mm x 10 mm x 10 mm), hexagons with a height of 6.3 mm and a width across flats of 13 mm), implants with a cylindrical center hole (all grade 5 titanium, Thyssen-Krupp, Germany) and inflow cannulas with a conical center hole (Produced by selective laser melting, provided by Kai von Petersdorff-Campen of the Product Development Group Zurich [46]) (see table 5.1).

Table 5.1: List of sample types used for the wax-disc and nanostructure etching route. The cubes were used for general testing, the hexagons for general testing and for all leak detection tests.

Sample Type	Wax-Disc Route	Nanostructure Etching
Cubes	X	
Hexagons		X
Implants	X	X
Inflow Cannulas		X

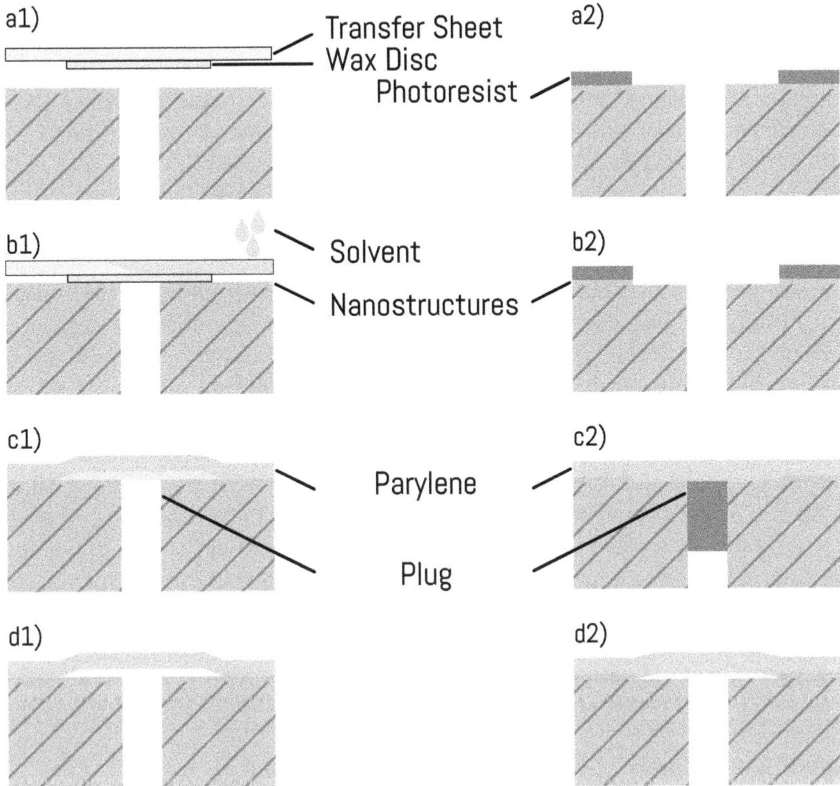

Figure 5.2: Process flow for wax-patch MSD fabrication (left) and Nanostructure patterning (right). Left: a1) After the flat wax disc is produced on a transfer sheet, the disc is pressed against the nanostructures, covering the pressure transmission channel. b1) Soaking the transfer sheet in solvent cause it to release the wax disc. c1) Parylene is coated over the nanostructures and wax disc. d1) the wax disc is dissolved and the MSD released. Right: a2) Photoresist is patterned to expose a MSD shaped area of the nanostructures around the pressure transmission channel. b2) The exposed area is etched to remove the nanostructures. c2) After filling the pressure transmission channel with a scrificial plug, parylene is coated. d2) The plug is dissolved and the low adhesion of parylene to titanium allows for the MSD to be released with little air pressure.

All surfaces where later an MSD would be created were first polished with sanding paper (grit: 1200 and 2400) and then cleaned in acetone, then isopropyl alcohol, and finally water in an ultrasonic bath. The samples were then placed in Teflon cups (50 mL) and NaOH (1 M) was added until the total volume of samples and NaOH reached 32 mL. For the implants the concentration was increased to 1.2 M to maintain the same NaOH content to titanium surface area used in [40]. For the cubes, seven were placed in each Teflon cup, for the hexagons four per cup, and the implants and inflow cannulas were placed into the cups individually. The cups were then closed and placed in steel cannisters and placed in a preheated oven at 180°C for 6 h. After removal from the oven, the cannisters were allowed to cool down for 2 h in ambient air before cooling with running tap water. After removal from the Teflon cups, the samples were placed in 2 subsequent DI-water baths for 10 min each before placing them in 0.5 mM HCl at 40°C for 24 h. The samples were then rinsed in DI-Water and blow-dried using pressurized air. Finally the samples were placed in a furnace. The furnace was set to heat up to 400°C over the course of 80 min, then hold the temperature for 1 h before cooling down again over the course of 200 min.

For the wax disc transfer route, beewax patches (CREATEC trend-design-GmbH, Germany) of different shapes with thicknesses in the range of 10 µm to 20 µm were prepared for transfer as follows: In a first step, transfer sheets (3652, Avery-Zweckform, Canada) were pressed between two polished aluminium plates in a hot-press with 10 t at 135°C for 10 min each to flatten their surface topography.

In a second step, the wax was pressed to thin sheets with a maximum thickness of 40 µm by repeated pressing and slicing cycles. For this, thick pieces of wax were sandwiched between two transfer sheets. This assembly was then placed in a hot press, using polished aluminium plates on top and under the sandwich to provide a flat surface during the pressing step. After applying 10 t at 35°C for 10 min, the sandwiches were allowed to cool down before removing the flattened wax from the sandwich. The resulting wax sheet was then cut into stripes of approximately 4 mm width. These stripes were then again placed between two transfer paper sheets and pressed. This cycle was repeated until a maximum thickness of around 30 µm to 40 µm was achieved. The thickness was verified by white light interferometer (WLI).

In a third step, laser-cut negative paper masks of the desired final wax-patch-shape were added to the sandwich (transfer paper, wax sheet, mask, transfer paper). This new sandwich was again placed in the hot-press, applying 2 t at 35°C for 10 min. Immediate removal of the mask, without cooling resulted in patches of the desired shape. To further reduce the thickness of the patches, a pressing step without mask was executed using 10 t at 35°C for 10 min before repeating the patterning step until the thickness of the patches reached thicknesses of 10 µm to 20 µm.

Before transfer, the transfer paper was cut into smaller pieces, each containing a single patch. The patch was then firmly pressed against the titanium nanostructures, using a stamp fitting the shape of the titanium sample (flat for cubes and curved for the implants) (fig 5.2 a1).

Release of the wax patch from the transfer sheet was induced by adding drops of acetone to the back side of the transfer sheet and waiting until the sheet released itself without manual help (fig 5.2 b1).

The titanium samples with wax sheets on them were then warmed up in an oven at 55°C just long enough for the edges of the patch to slightly melt in an effort to create a smoother border of the MSD.

The prepared samples were coated with Parylene-C (P6, Diener Electronics, Germany), using 30 g of Parylene precursor (fig 5.2 c1). The evaporation chamber's temperature was automatically feedback controlled to maintain 30 µbar (3 Pa) in the deposition chamber and limited to 170°C. The pyrolysis tube was set to 720°C and the deposition chamber was heated to 40°C. Before starting the process, the chamber was evacuated to pressures below 10 µbar (1 Pa) and the process was automatically terminated after the precursor was fully consumed. Parylene layer thickness was measured using the WLI on a separate glass-slide placed in the deposition chamber along with the samples.

The sacrificial wax patch was dissolved by submerging the samples in heptane at 40°C (fig 5.2 d1). Trapped air bubbles in the pressure transmission channel were manually removed using a blunt stick to accelerate the wax dissolution and prevent damage to the MSD.

For the nanostructure etch route, nanostructured samples were dip coated in photoresist (AZ 4562, Merck Performance Materials GmbH, Germany)(INFO) and prebaked for 2 h at 800°C. Laser-cut polyimide masks (fig. 5.3 a: mask for implants) were placed on the samples or inside the implants (fig. 5.3 b) before illumination using a UV mask aligner (MABA6, Suess Microtec, Germany) and, for the implants to reach the inner side walls, a 45° mirror (fig. 5.3 c), for 60 s. The photoresist was then developed in AZ 400 K diluted 1:4 with DI water for 2 min 30 s. After rinsing (fig. 5.3 d) and drying, the samples were post-baked for 2 h at 1100°C (fig 5.2 a2). The exposed areas were etched using hydrofluoric acid (48 % Sigma-Aldrich, USA) diluted 1:100 (fig 5.2 b2). The samples were placed in the acid until bubble formation was observed in the exposed areas and kept there for an additional 90 s, 120 s, 150 s, and 200 s for the hexagonal samples and 105 s for the inflow cannulae and implants. Then all samples were immediately rinsed in two subsequent DI-water baths before activating the quick-dump-rinser and blow-drying them with pressurized air. Stripping was done in acetone for 10 min in an ultrasonic bath and subsequent rinsing steps were performed with IPA and DI-Water. The MSD beds in the implants were additionally

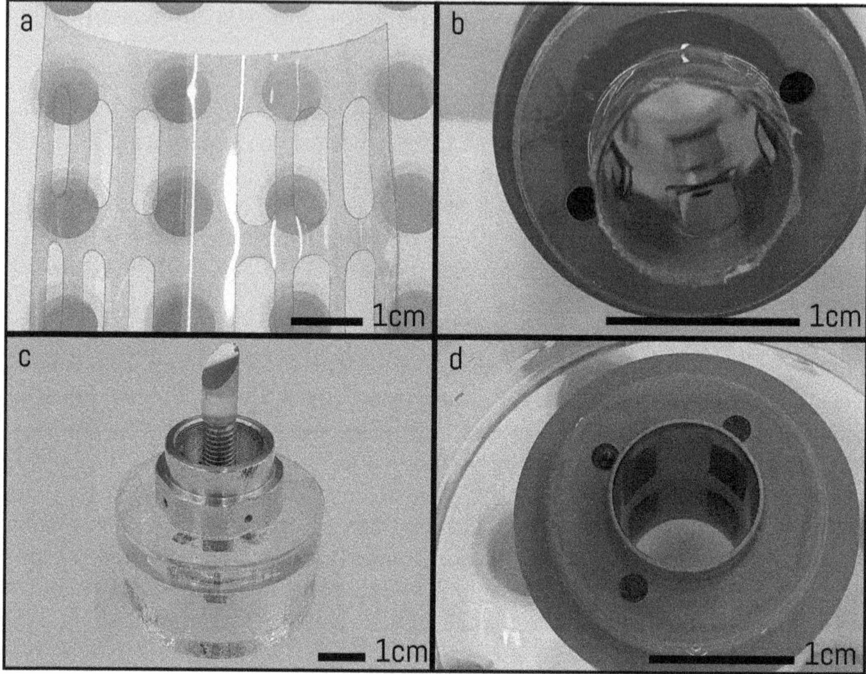

Figure 5.3: Photographic images of the photolithography process used before the etching of the nanostructures. a) the mask used to expose the photoresist to UV. The left group of MSD shaped cut-outs is the shape of the MSD. b) a rolled up mask inside an implant body. c) Implant holder with 45° mirror. d) Implant with developed photoresist. The areas to be etched are exposed.

cleaned with a 2400 gritt sanding paper, passing two times using very light pressure to remove residues from the etching process.

The etched depth was measured using the WLI and observed using a scanning electron microscope (Nova NanoSEM 450, FEI/Thermo Fisher Scientific USA).

After metalization (see ch. 5.3) for the electrical feedthrough, and plugging of the pressure transmission channel for all samples (see ch. 5.2) (fig. 5.2 c1), Parylene coating was performed as described above.

Release of the MSD was achieved by applying pressurized air of at least 0.5 bar (50 kPa) in the pressure transmission channel, after dissolving the plug (fig 5.2 d1).

5.1.3 Results & Discussion

The nanostructure growth process was found to result in the desired petal-like structures for cubes and hexagons (Fig. 5.4, a,b). The initial concentration resulted in poorly developed structures on implants. The concentration was increased from 1 M NaOH to 1.2 M NaOH to achieve the same NaOH content to titanium surface ratio for the implants as it was for the cubes. This step improved the nanostructure development to some extent even if some optical variation was still observable among the implants and inflow cannulas (Fig. 5.4, c,d vs. e,f). As no delamination of the Parylene layer outside of the desired area was observed during the MSD release, the interlocking strength was deemed sufficient and the nanostructure growth process was not further investigated.

For the wax patch method, no problems in the initial pressing and slicing steps were observed. The thick layers remained easy to handle and slice and the slicing lead to more uniform layer thicknesses with each cycle. When reaching a thickness of around 30 µm to 40 µm the adhesion to the transfer sheet would become stronger then the strength of the wax layer, causing tearing. Peeling off the wax layers would become unfeasible both with and without solvent. This however enabled the patterning by use of wax absorbing mask sheets. Pressing the mask into the wax layer would result in the absorption of the wax into the mask, creating strong adhesion of the layer. Peeling off the mask would then cause the wax layer to tear along the borders of the MSD shaped holes in the mask, leaving only the shaped wax patches on the transfer sheet (Fig. 5.5). This step worked remarkably well. However the variation of thickness of the wax layer sometimes caused wax patches to be removed from the transfer sheet along with the mask, where the wax layer was thickest. It was also observed that the adhesion of the wax layer to the transfer sheet increased with every use, even if the sheets were removed on alternating sides after each step. The wax patches on finished transfer sheets still showed significant variation in thickness, causing 40 % of the patches to be discarded (Fig. 5.6), reducing the yield. Furthermore, the tearing of the wax layer along the edges of the patches caused these edges to become slight frayed. Transfer of the wax patches to the nanostructured surfaces worked well even if occasionally the patch would detach from the sample instead of the transfer sheet. This gentle method enabled the transfer of wax patches down to 10 µm even across pressure transmission channel without support (e.g.: such as first plugging the channel). The frayed borders of the wax patches remained even after transfer (Fig. 5.7), necessitating a short curing step. The melting of the frayed edges into a clean border was easily observable and a viable solution for single MSD devices and resulted in clean Parylene MSDs after coating (Fig. 5.8). For multi MSD devices, this method became inapplicable as the onset of smoothing occured at different times for different MSDs and continued heat exposure after the onset would cause the

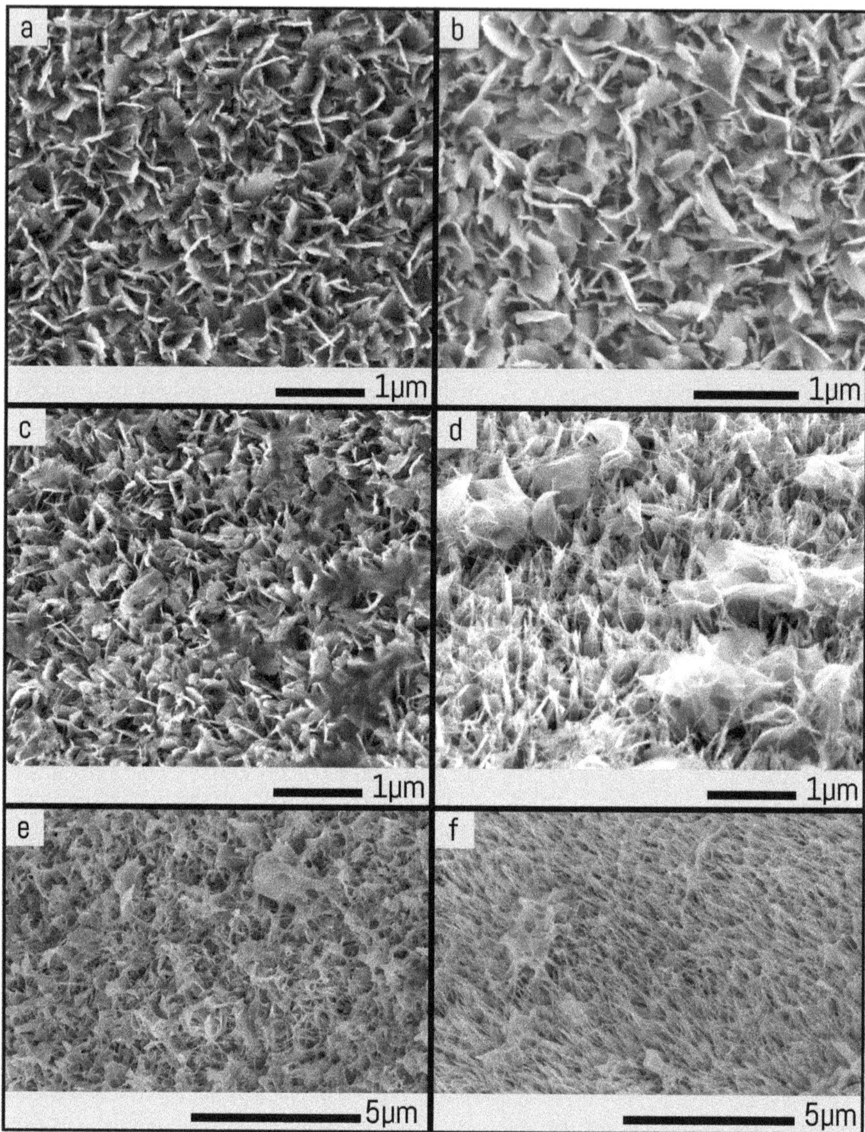

Figure 5.4: SEM images of nanostructures. (a,b): grown on flat samples (cube, hexagon respectively), (c): grown on the outside of an implant (30° angle), (d): on the inside of an implant (45° angle) (e,f): inflow cannulas. The shape of nanostructures ranged from petal-like (a) to near pure needle-forest-like (f). Image (b) produced by Ian Hutter.

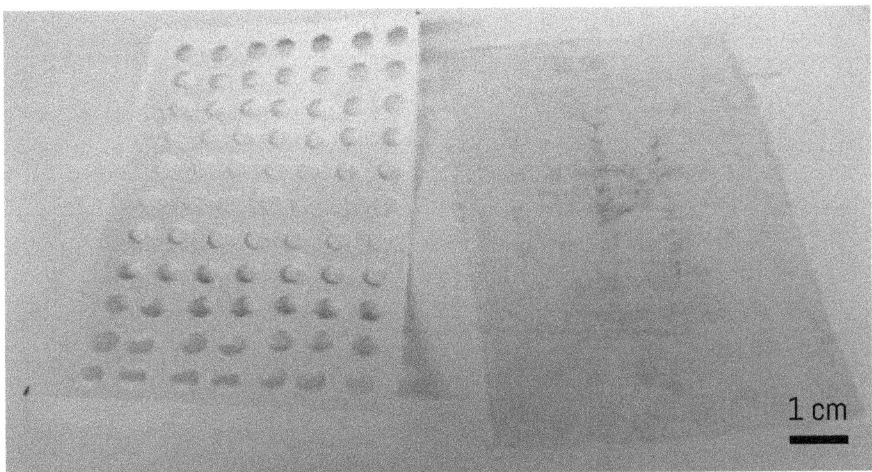

Figure 5.5: Photographic image of the paper mask used to absorb excess wax and shape the discs (left) and the transfer sheet, with the finished wax discs (right).

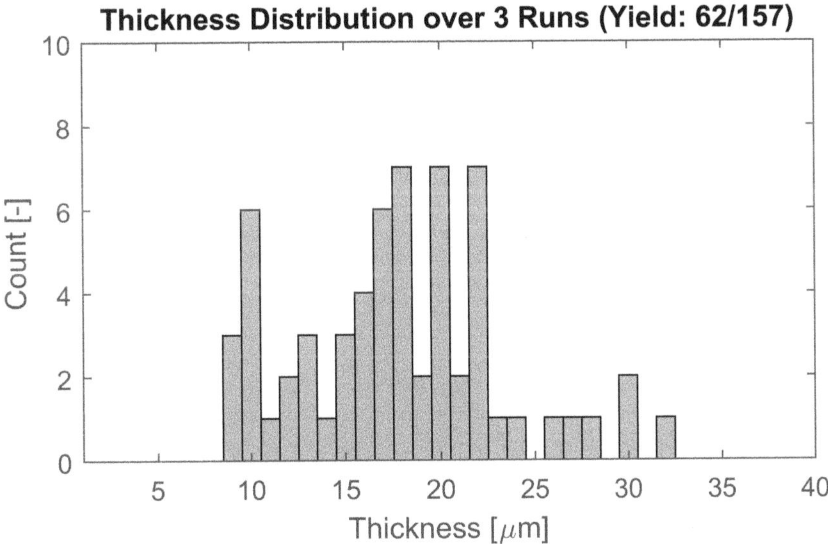

Figure 5.6: Histogram of the thickness of the wax discs for 3 full runs. Less than half the discs remained undamaged to the end and only a small amount of discs reached the optimal target thickness of 10 µm.

part of the wax patch covering the pressure transmission channel to slowly move into the channel, breaking the smooth surface of the patch and later MSD. Using this method in combination with a plunging of the pressure

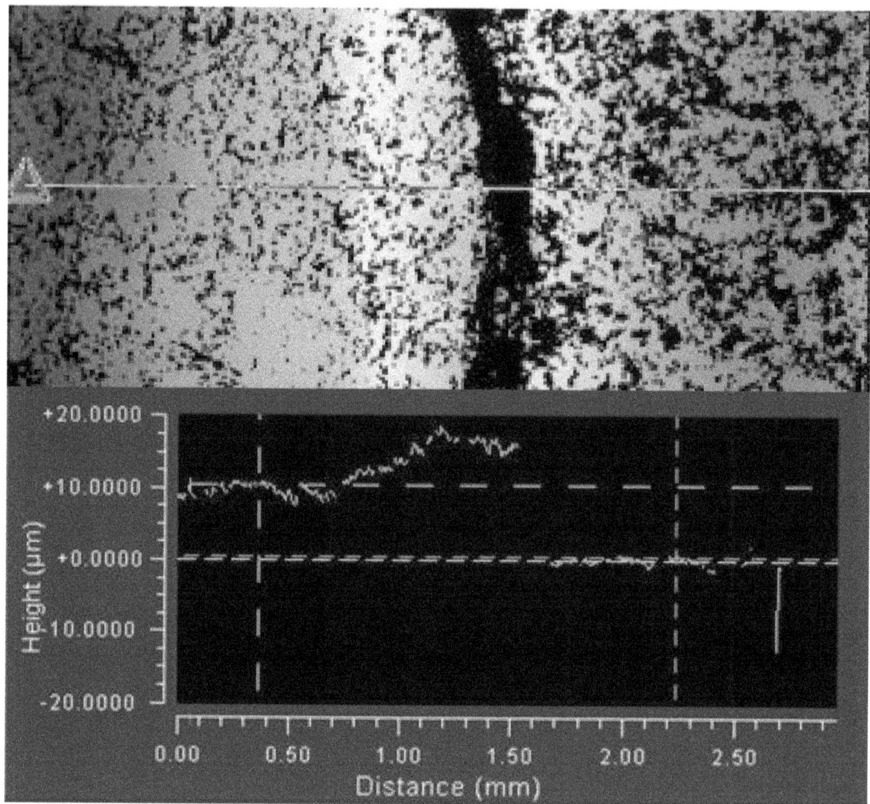

Figure 5.7: Surface profile of the edge of a wax disc after transfer, recorded by WLI. The edge is higher than the rest of the patch, likely due to local delamination or imperfect transfer.

transmission channel might resolve this problem but was not attempted. Complete release of the MSDs by dissolution of the wax patch with heptane posed no problems. In samples produced with this method, it was observed that after further processing steps, which included heating of the sample, the MSDs would become stuck to the titanium. A potential explanation could be the remaining nanostructures underneath the MSD which might have rejoined themselves with the MSD when exceeding its glass transition temperature and pressing the MSD against the nanostructures.

For the etching method (fig. 5.9), etch depth measurements of the MSD bed showed a much better correlation with the etching time from bubble onset than with the total exposure time to HF (Fig 5.10). No apparent connection between production run or container in which the nanostructures were grown and the time to bubble formation was observed (Fig 5.11). For each MSD

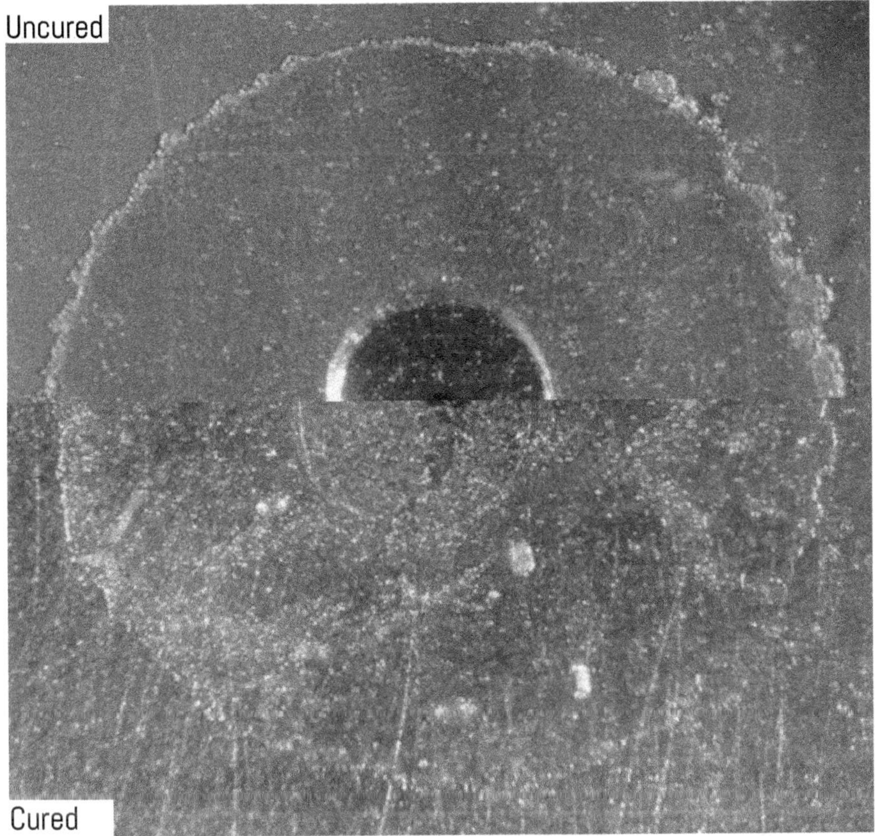

Figure 5.8: Optical microscope image of a Parylene MSD (d = 5 mm) produced on an uncured (top) and cured (bottom) wax disc. The MSD produced on the uncured disc shows a clear border, whereas the border of the MSD in the bottom image are nearly invisible

bed, 3 measurements were taken and the distribution relative to the average value is shown in Figure 5.11. There are multiple factors potentially affecting the end result, such as wetting, photoresist residues, nanostructure and oxide thickness and variation in bubble detection by the operator. The last factor could at least to some extent explain the average etch depth variation seen in figure 5.10, right and is probably also a partial cause for the spread in time to first bubble seen in figure 5.11, left. The spread in time to first bubble is larger than the deviation amongst the average times to first bubbles per production batch/canister, indicating that varying production factors among the canisters are not the cause for the large spread.

Wetting could be a potential explanation due to the complex surface struc-

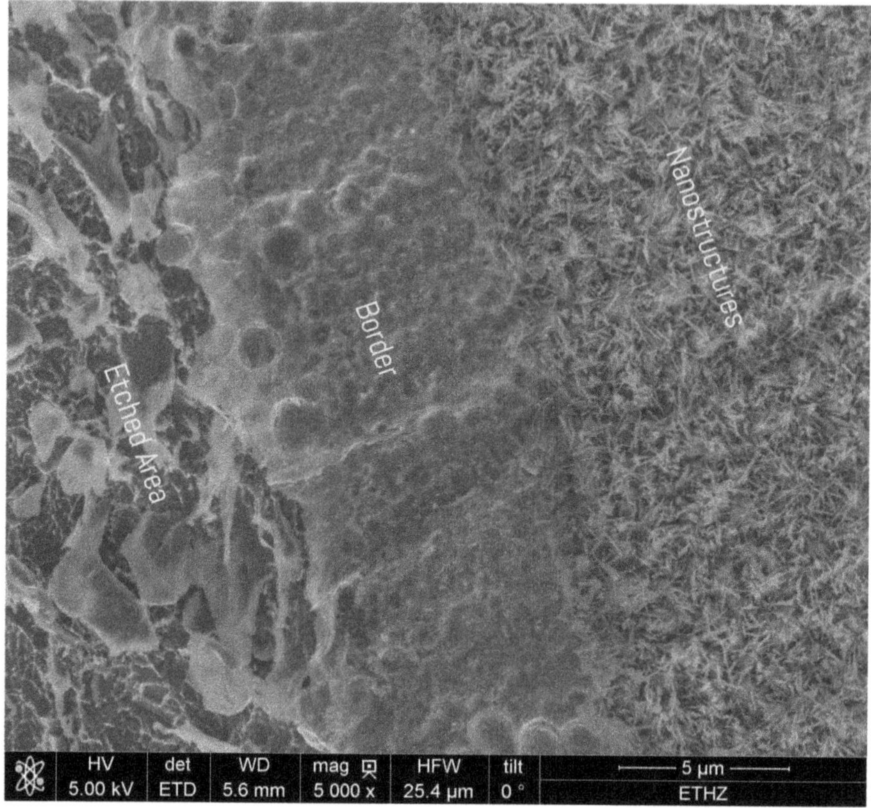

Figure 5.9: SEM image of the border region of the etched area. The etched (left) transitional (middle) and un-etched area are visible.

ture. Pre-wetting with application of vacuum could help remove gas pockets in the structure and allow the chemical reaction to start more equally. It was assumed that formation of bubbles indicated the onset of the reaction between HF and pure titanium and is a result of the increased hydrogen formation in the absence of oxygen available during the etching of titanium oxide. Additionally, remaining trapped gaseous oxygen might also play a role here.

However, the achieved spread in etching depth was deemed sufficiently precise for the goal of completely removing the nanostructures and etching less than half the thickness of the MSD (20 µm) into the titanium body. The etching process was thus not investigated further and translated to the implants and inflow cannulae.

Delamination of the MSDs in the inflow cannulae occurred at around

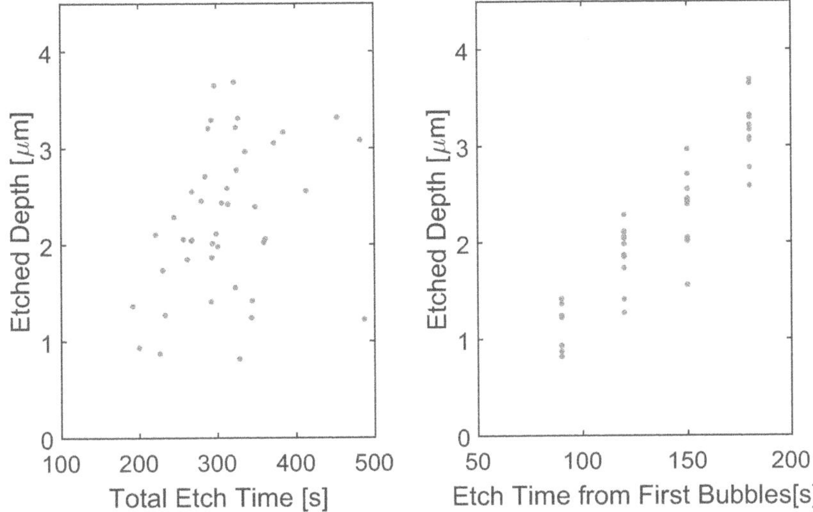

Figure 5.10: Etched depth for multiple MSD beds as function of the total immersion time (left) and the time recorded from the onset of the first bubbles (right). The latter offers a much better prediction of the resulting etched depth. Data acquired by Ian Hutter

1 bar (100 kPa) for half the MSDs. For the other half only partial delamination was achieved even at pressures up to 2.5 bar (250 kPa). For the implants delamination occurred below 1 bar (100 kPa) for all MSDs. This difference is attributed to the removal of residues visible in the etched area in figure 5.12, by cleaning after etching. It should be noted, that these residues were not observed in the first implant (fig. 5.13) used to verify the etching parameters and full delamination was achieved without the added manual cleaning of the membrane bed. Optimization of the etching process for implants and cannulae should be considered to eliminate the tedious cleaning of the MSD bed. Nevertheless, the etching route produced significantly smoother Parylene-coating to MSD border areas in implants and cannulae, mostly due to the afore mentioned difficulties with the curing step in the wax disc route (fig. 5.14).

5.1.4 Conclusion

The wax patch process achieved its target to block Parylene-nanostructure anchoring in defined areas while retaining a smooth Parylene coating. However, the time consuming and labour intensive series of thickness measuring and flattening as well as the difficult to control smoothening step before coating rendered this method impractical for a controllable implant produc-

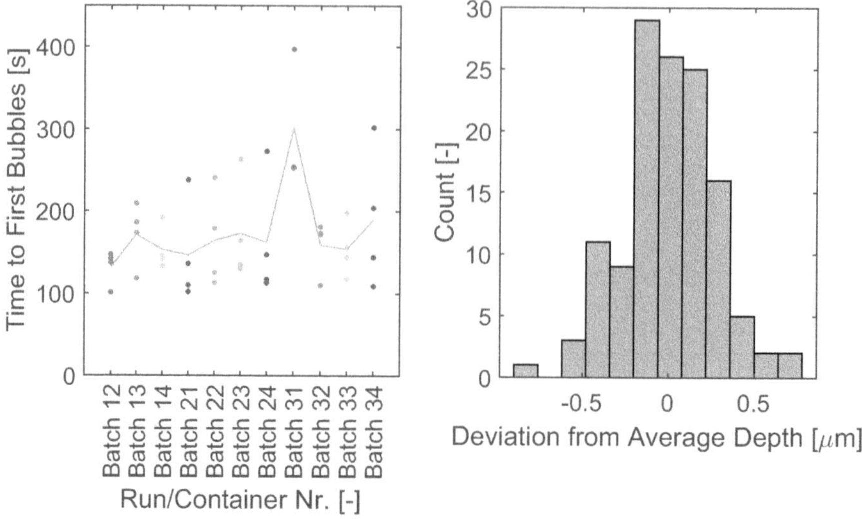

Figure 5.11: Left: Time from start of immersion in etchant until the appearance of the first bubble, for each production batch. The line shows the average for each batch. No clear difference between the batches is visible. Right: Etch depth deviation distribution from the group average (group is defined by the etch time after bubbles, see fig. 5.10, right) for all samples. Data acquired by Ian Hutter

tion with the tools available. If a solution could be found to easily produce thin wax layers of uniform thickness in the 10 µm range on transfer sheets, this method would become viable again. It is also suggested here to use this method in combination with the plugging of the transfer channel to allow taking full advantage of the smoothening happening in the final curing step.

The etching path achieved its target to create an area of controlled easy delamination for MSD formation with a depth of less than half the MSD size. With exception of the illumination step with the UV light source used here all steps are highly parallelizable. However, that step could be accelerated by using an insertable radiation source. This method proved being more reliable and precise, produced smoother MSD borders and achieved lower MSD border heights than the wax patch method and was therefore chosen for the production of the inflow cannulas and final implant batch.

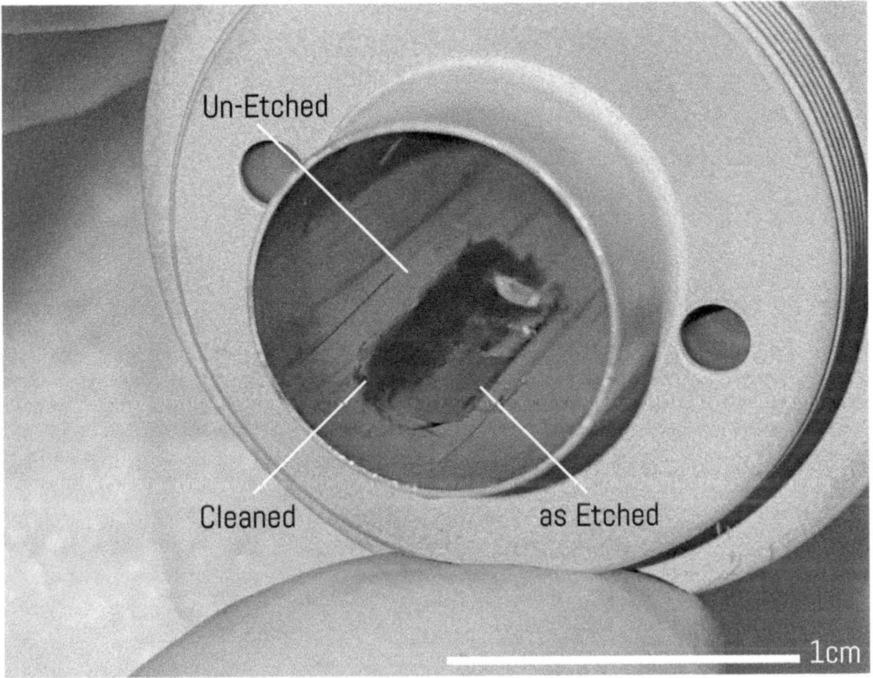

Figure 5.12: Photographic Image of an MSD bed with the left side cleaned and the right as obtained after the etching process. Unlike in the pilot sample, etching did not result in a cleanly etched surface and manual wiping was required to obtain a surface as seen in fig. 5.13.

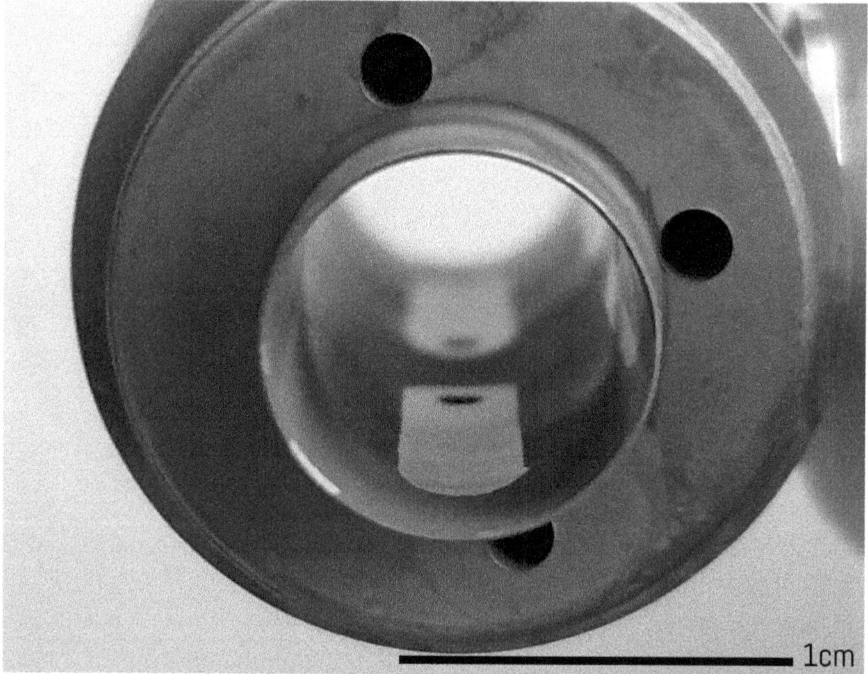

Figure 5.13: Photographic image of the pilot implant after etching and stripping of the photoresist. The clean shiny surface is the etched area.

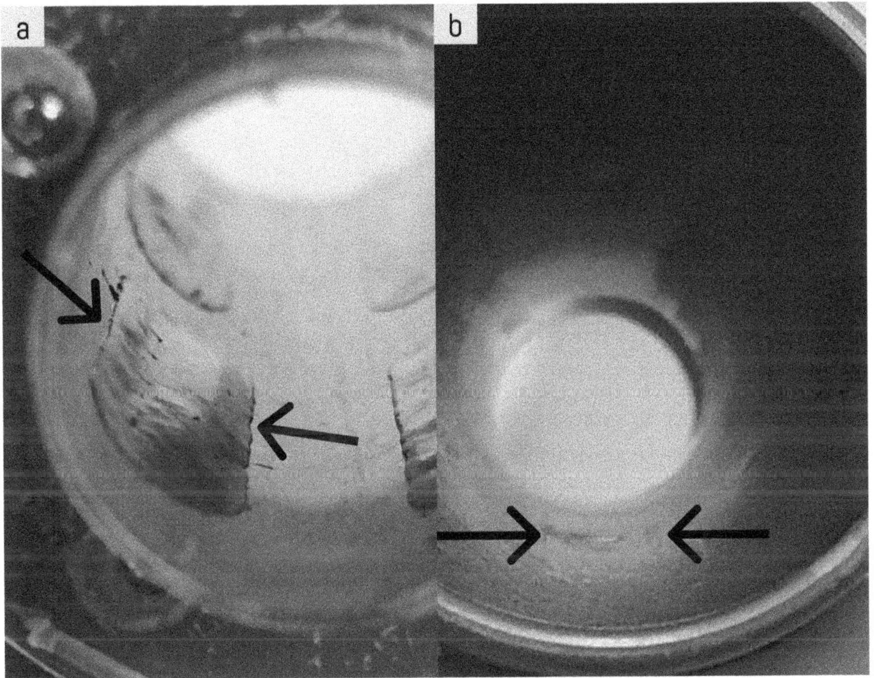

Figure 5.14: Photographic Images of MSDs produces with the wax-patch route (a) and etch route (b). The border of the MSD can clearly be seen in (a) and becomes nearly invisible in (b).

5.2 Channel Plug

A study exploring multiple alternative sacrificial materials for the channel plug with alternative solidification routes, better adhesive properties to titanium but not to the plate (see fig. 5.15), ease of handling, and better ductility was performed by Paula Martin [47]. The best results were finally obtained by compressing powder sugar inside the channel (fig. 5.15), thus eliminating the liquid to solid transition from the process.

5.2.1 Materials & Methods

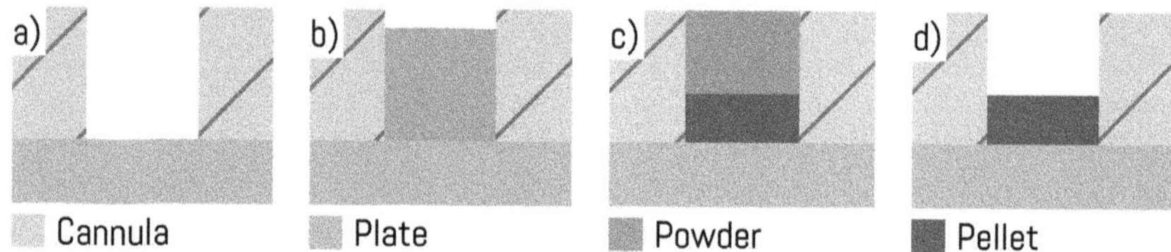

Figure 5.15: Schematic of the sacrificial plug formation in the pressure transmission channel, using the sugar compression method.

In the case of flat samples, a flat, polished plate (silver steel) was pressed against the sample, covering the pressure transmission channel. For the implants and cannulae a counter plate matching the curvature of either sample was used (see fig. 5.16). Powder sugar was filled into the pressure transmission channel from the other side and compressed using a steel rod with the same diameter as the channel using a tensile testing station (5848 Micro Tester, Instron, USA). Compressive Forces in the range of 0.3 kN to 2 kN were applied. The resulting sugar surface as well as the used plate was observed by microscopy and WLI.

5.2.2 Results & Discussion

Figure 5.17 shows a sugar plug in an implant, before Parylene coating. Figure 5.18 shows a WLI image and surface profile of a pellet produced by this method using 500 N. While nearly perfectly flat, the compression was not sufficient across the whole surface. Very high forces on the other hand resulted in protrusion of the plug up to 30 µm from the surface and plastic deformation of the plate. A compromise between compression and protrusion was found at 850 N, resulting in stable plugs with peak protrusion below 10 µm. The application of vacuum had no observable effect on the pellets.

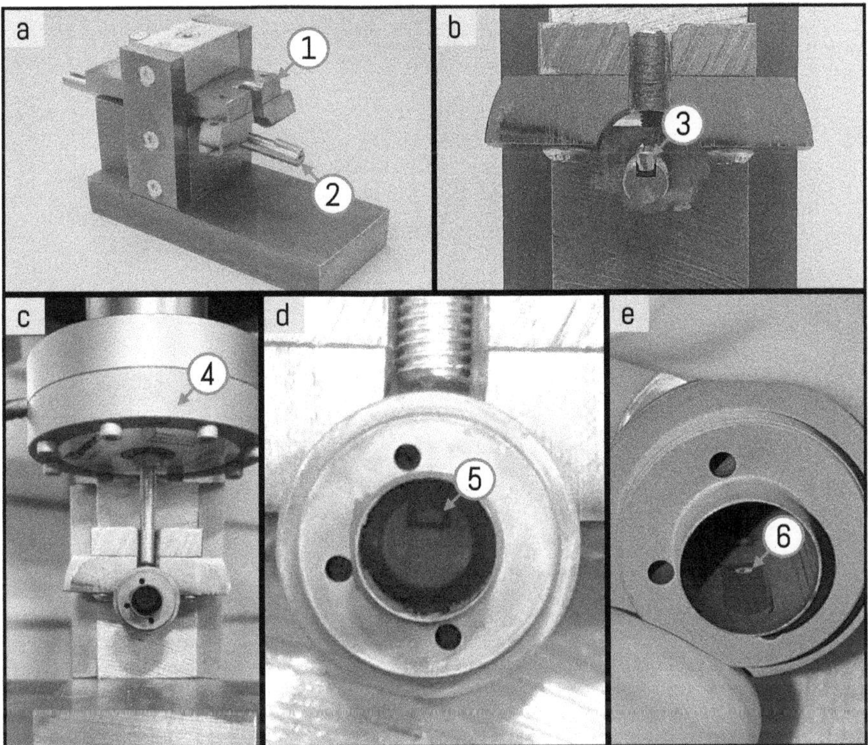

Figure 5.16: Photographic images if the sugar plug process. a) Implant holder with clamp (1) and slide-able rod (2). b) Frontal view with the replaceable counter plate (3) with matched radius to the implant's inner surface. c) Implant holder with mounted implant during the sugar plug compression step, with the force measurement device (4). d) Close-up view of the mounted implant with the replaceable counter plate pressed against the inner surface of the implant during the sugar plug compression step. e) Sugar plug in pressure transmission channel after compression.

The indentations in the plates under higher forces indicate that the limiting factor was its hardness. This suggests that using superhard materials such as ceramics could result in even flatter and more stable compressed pellets. It should be noted that, unlike the previously suggested wax process, this approach is serial. This was not considered a disadvantage for the production of a small implant series due to its much quicker execution, high reliability and the option to remake a single plug, while leaving others in place.

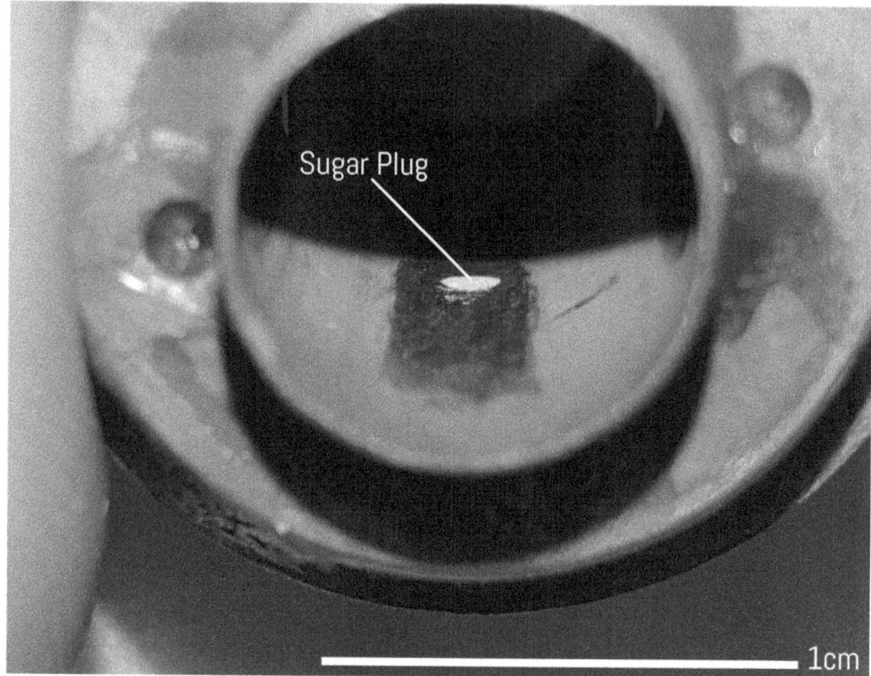

Figure 5.17: Photographic image of an implant with sugar plug. The difference in color from fig. 5.13 and fig. 5.12 is due to different lighting and lighting angles.

5.2.3 Conclusion

A parameter set for the production of compressed sugar plugs with sufficient stability and low protrusion was found and deemed sufficient for the scope of this work. This process was chosen over the previously suggested wax processes due to its high reliably and economic time cost and the ability to individually remake single plugs.

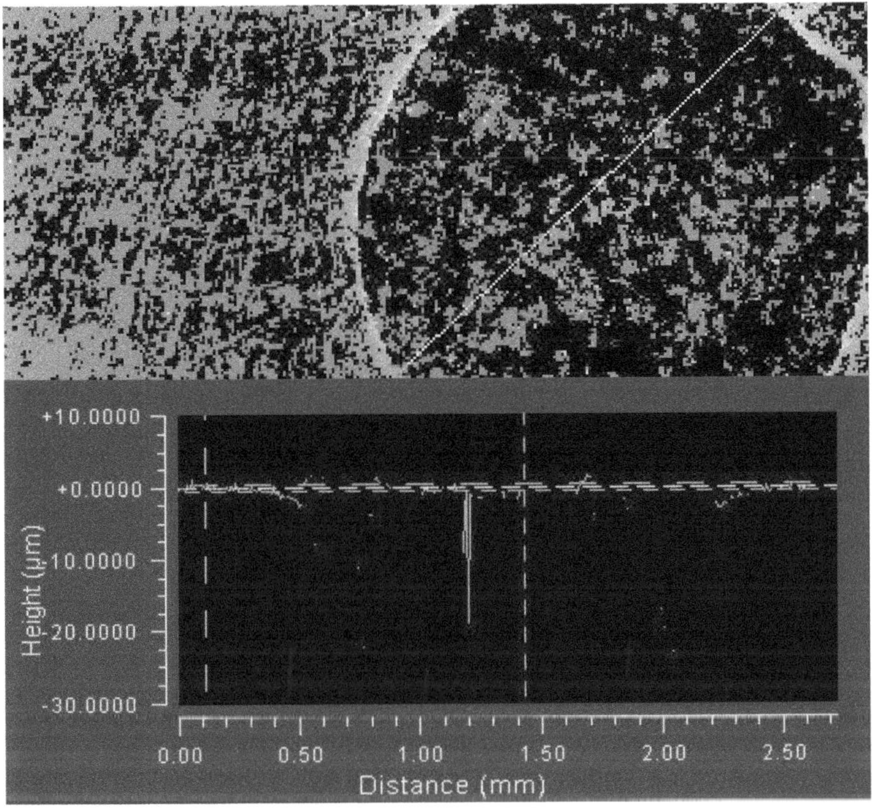

Figure 5.18: WLI surface profile image of a sacrificial compressed sugar plug in the pressure transmission channel of a flat sample.

5.3 Electrical Feedthrough

The electrical feed through allows electronic communication with an encapsulated sensor while sealing the pressure transmission oil inside.

5.3.1 Materials & Methods

To enable soldering to the titanium bodies of the implants and inflow cannulae, 30 nm Ti, 100 nm Ni, 300 nm Cu, and 150 nm Au were evaporated onto the target surfaces (fig. 5.19) by Martin Kloeckner of the Laboratory Support Group (D-PHYS, ETHZ). For this, the surface roughness of the target surfaces was increased using a 400 gritt sanding paper. After washing the implant and IC bodies in Acetone, IPA and water, an in-situ

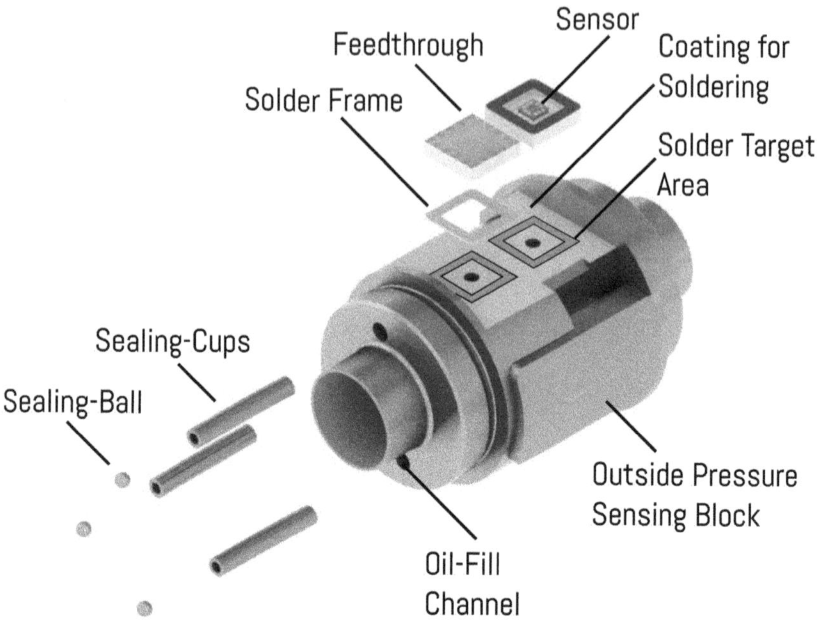

Figure 5.19: Exploded view of the implant with the target area for soldering of the electrical feedthrough, the solder material frame, and the sensor inside the package used as electrical feedthrough.

vacuum-baking step at 500°C and over night cooling step was executed before using a rotating suspension for homogeneous layer evaporation. Packages (P18LCC120S1, Kyocera, Japan) were prepared by soldering a mini PCB to their bottom (fig. 5.20 a), connecting the mini-PCB pads to the pads of the package by wire bonding (fig. 5.20 b), soldering the sensor (LPS22HB, STMicroelectronics, Switzerland) onto the mini PCB and filling the area around the sensor with CTE matched protective polymer mass (Epo-TEK OG 116-31, Epoxy Technology, Switzerland) to insulate the wire bonds (fig. 5.20 c). The prepared packages were then soldered to larger PCBs for signal distribution. The prepared package assemblies were then pressed against the implant bodies with a precut In48Sn solder frame (Indalloy 1E, Indium Corporation, USA) in-between, using a suspension system (fig. 5.21) applying 2 N. Two drops of flux (5 RMA-RC, Indium Corporation, USA) were added to the solder frame and the assembly placed in an oven (Heraeus drying cabinet, Heraeus Group, Switzerland) at 40°C. After evacuation, the oven was refilled with N_2. The oven was then heated to 160°C over the course of around 12 minutes and the temperature kept there for 10 min, before allowing the oven to cool down over night (fig. 5.20 d).

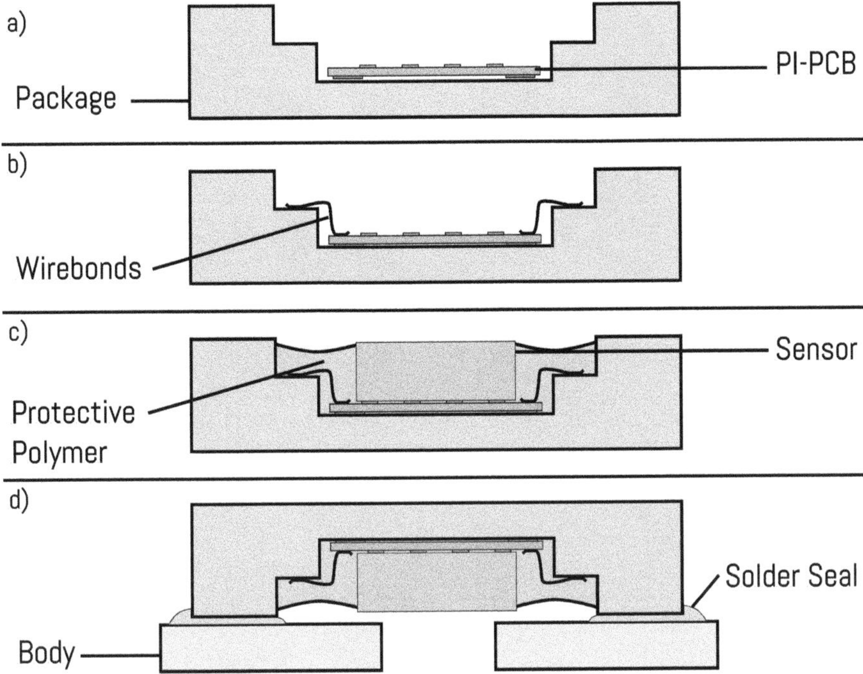

Figure 5.20: Schematic of the workflow for the electrical feedthrough. a) Soldering the polyimide PCB onto the floor of the package. b) Connecting the PI-PCB to the pads of the package by wirebonding. c) Soldering the sensor to the PI-PCB and adding the protective polymer mass. d) Low temperature soldering of the assembly to the implant covering the pressure transmission channel.

5.3.2 Results & Discussion

The final Ti/Ni/Cu/Au stack was suggested by Martin Kloeckner and Sandro Tiegermann of the Laboratory Support Group (D-PHYS, ETHZ). For the adhesion-layer, Ti was chosen over Cr due to its match with the substrate material. The Ni layer was thought to serve as a diffusion barrier, Cu as the solder target and Au as an oxidation protection layer, that would be completely dissolved during the electrical feedthrough soldering.

Samples with polished target surfaces displayed large, film-like delamination of the evaporated layers exceeding areas directly exposed to stress. This was not observed for samples with increased surface roughness, possibly due to local confinement of the delamination propagation by the non flat surface. The in-situ vacuum-baking step was found to further significantly improve the adhesion of the evaporated layers, possibly by removing residual con-

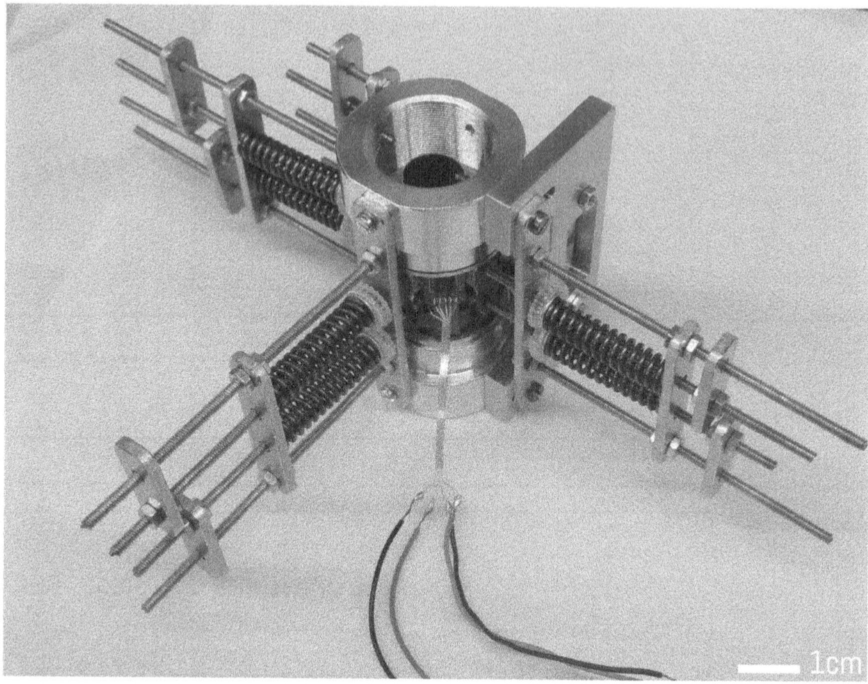

Figure 5.21: Photographic image of implant prepared for solder sealing of the packages to the implant's surface. The spring regulate the force with which the packages are pressed against the implant.

taminations. Higher temperatures as well as fast heating/cooling rates were found to damage the nanostructures by melting and cracking respectively and therefore avoided for the device production. An implant body with the applied metalization is visible in figure 5.22.

The use of packages as electrical feedthrough was chosen as they combine rigidity, a target surface to solder to and are readily available in a large variety of shapes and sizes. Figure 5.23 shows an assembled package attached to a PCB, without the CTE matched protective polymer mass and triple wirebonding per pad connection. A custom made ceramic PCB would have drastically reduced the complexity and failure rate of the sub-assembly. The most common failure modes were found to be damaged wirebonds, incorrect or incomplete reflow soldering of the sensor to the mini PCB and accidental blocking of the sensor's own pressure transmission channels, by overflowing polymer mass. Different solder materials, and a wide range of process parameters were studied for this purpose by Roland Graf [44].

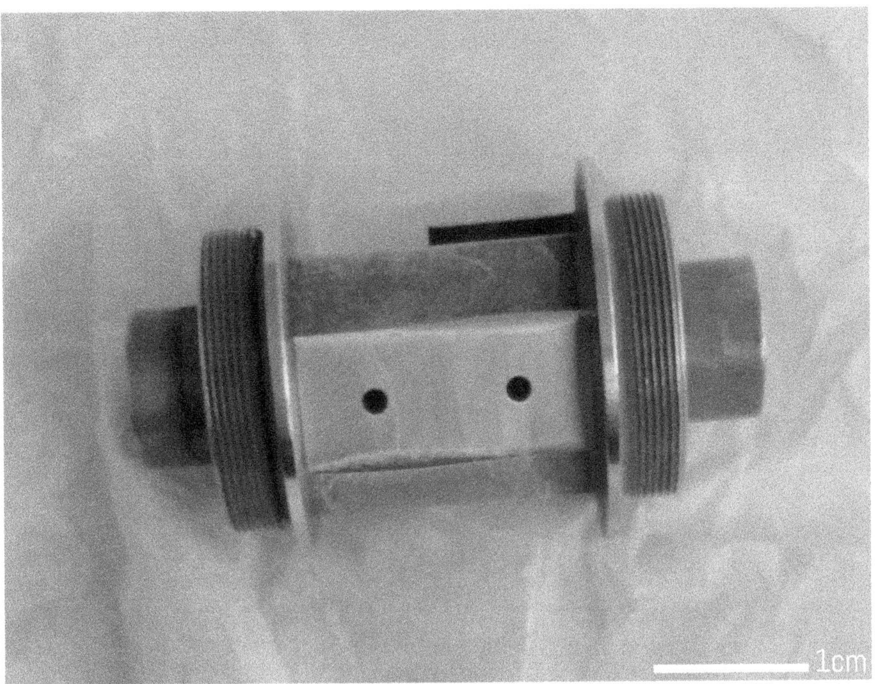

Figure 5.22: Photographic image of an implant after metalization for soldering.

5.3.3 Conclusion

The solder sealing process itself was found to produce reliable, leak free bonds, given proper metalization.

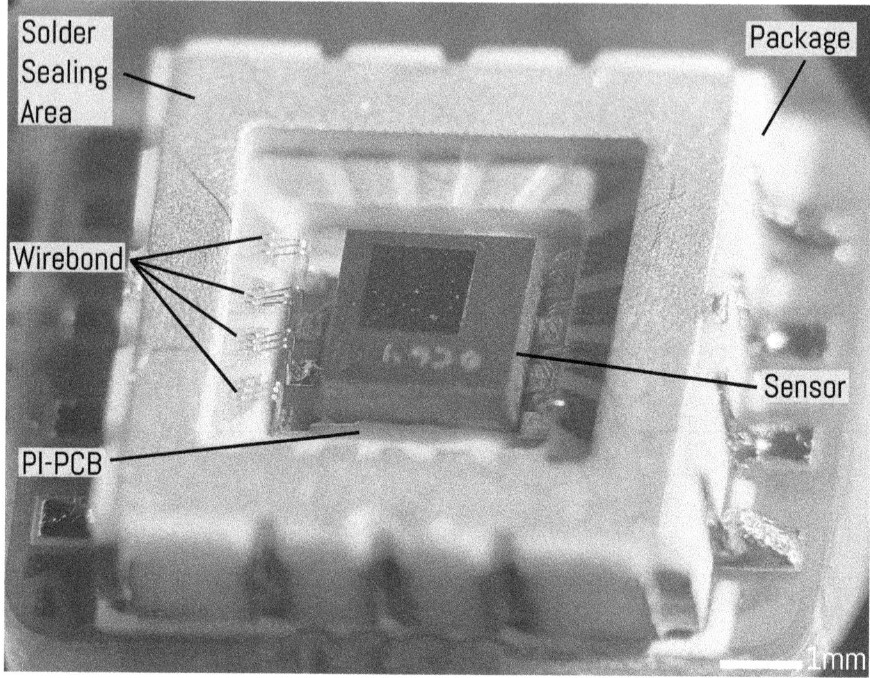

Figure 5.23: Photographic image of an electrical feedthrough assembly consisting of a ceramic package, a polyimide mini PCB, connected with 3 wirebonds per pad-pair and the sensor in the center.

5.4 Backside Sealing

The backside sealing closes the oil-fill channel in a last fabrication step, sealing the oil into the capsule. Commonly used ball-only seals, where a ball of slightly larger diameter than the oil-fill channel is pressed into the channel, push some amount of oil into the capsules, resulting in a small pressure increase. The volume of oil can roughly be estimated as the area of the channel, multiplied with the insertion depth of the ball at the diameter where sealing is achieved. In common applications, the MSD has a much larger diameter than the oil-fill channel and the injected oil thus causes only neglectable pressure increase inside the capsule. For the small MSD sizes, limited by the inflow cannula diameter and curvature, used in this work, this would result in a significant over-pressure after sealing and strong drift, due to the viscoelastic nature of the used MSD material. The used sealing approach in this work strongly reduces both post-assembly over-pressure as well as the resulting drift by minimizing the injected oil volume.

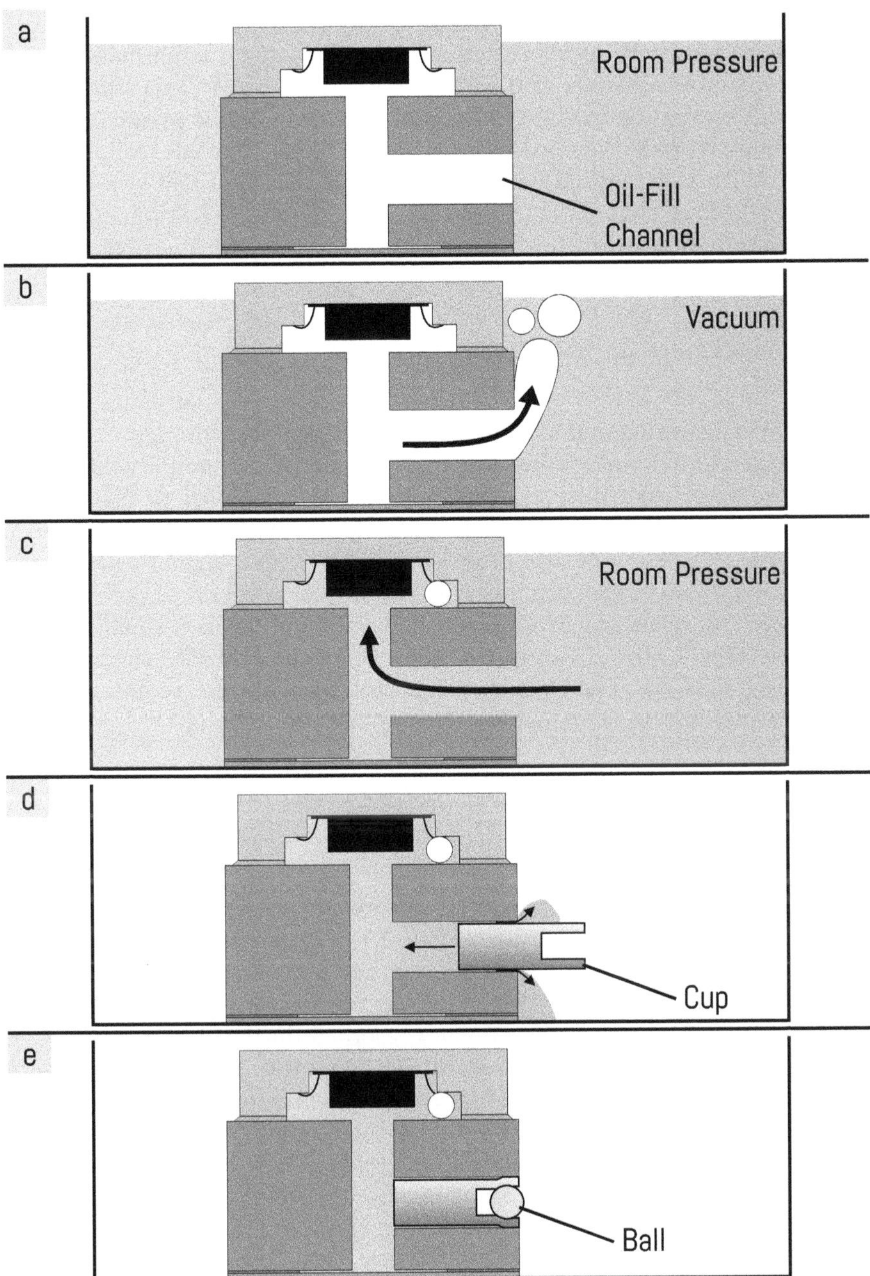

Figure 5.24: Schematic of the oil-fill and backside-sealing process. a) The capsule is submerged in oil. b) Vacuum is applied, expanding the trapped air in the capsule. Excess air leaves the capsule. c) Vacuum is released, compressing the trapped air and allowing oil to flood the capsule. d) The cup is placed in the oil-fill channel, displacing the oil inside the channel. e) The ball is pressed into the cup, expanding it and sealing the capsule.

This is achieved by first inserting a loosely fitted cup into the oil-fill channel, which displaces the oil inside the channel, only leaving a minuscule amount between the oil-fill channel wall and the outer cup wall. In this state excess oil can still escape the capsule. After stabilization a ball is pressed into the cup, pressing its walls outwards against the oil-filling channel, sealing off the capsule. With this method only the oil trapped in the small gap between cup and oil-filling channel is pressed into the capsule, resulting in a much lower pressure increase and drift, compared to a ball only solution.

5.4.1 Materials & Methods

After MSD fabrication and soldering of the electrical feedthrough and sensor testing, the devices were submerged in silicone oil (Bluesil FLD47 v 50, Elkem, Norway) (fig. 5.24, a). Vacuum was then applied to expand the air remaining inside the capsule (the unloaded vacuum chamber can reach 20 mbar (2 kPa)) (fig. 5.24, b). After 1 h, and gentle tapping of the devices to free trapped bubbles, the vacuum was released, allowing oil to flow into the capsules as the remaining trapped air collapses and forms a small residual air bubble (fig. 5.24, c). A cup was then slowly pushed into the oil-filling channel (fig. 5.24, d). The built up overpressure was allowed to decay, before pushing a ball into the cup, sealing the capsule (fig. 5.24, e).

5.4.2 Results & Discussion

Figure 5.25 shows a cross section of an assembled backside sealing. The steel ball presses the brass cup outwards against the titanium, creating a sealing area. The areas marked in read, represent the part of the gap between the cup and the oil-filling channel where oil was pressed into the capsule (downwards). Figure 5.26 shows the pressure recorded during the final assembly step by the enclosed sensor. The sensor initially measures ambient pressure (subtracted), then records multiple, rapidly decaying pressure peaks due to the insertion of the cup (fig.5.24 a/b). At nine minutes the ball is pressed into the cup (fig.5.24 c/d) and the capsule sealed. A small pressure increase without decay is recorded. The small spikes are caused by movement.

5.4.3 Conclusion

The ball-cup solution, as used in this work still produces a small overpressure inside the capsule, which is significantly smaller than a ball only sealing

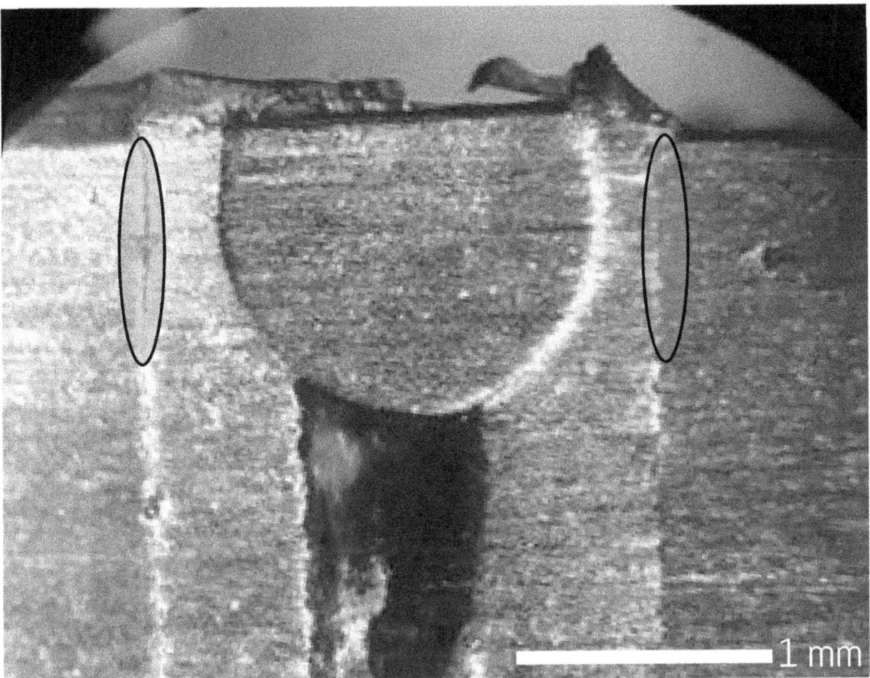

Figure 5.25: Microscopy image of the cross-section of a steel ball, pressed into a brass-cup in a mock filling channel. The deformation of the brass is visible and the ball entered the filling channel deeper than it's equator. The areas marked in red (oval) show the areas from where residual oil would be pushed downwards and into the capsule.

solution. Optimizing the cup to oil-filling channel fit could result in even small final overpressure by reducing the trapped oil volume at the cost of slower overpressure decay and longer assembly times. Increasing the wait time after cup insertion could further reduce the overall overpressure.

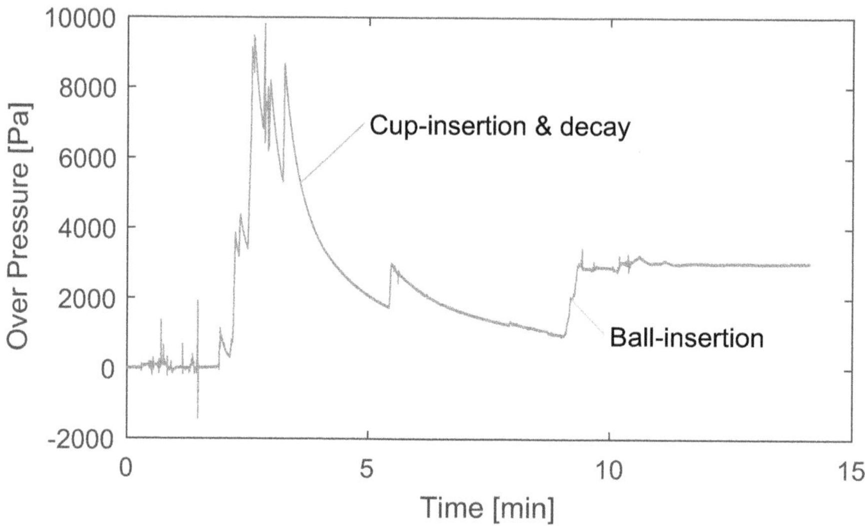

Figure 5.26: Recorded pressure during the final sealing process. The high peaks on the left occur during the insertion of the cup and decay quickly as the cup does not fully seal the capsule, but allow excess oil to escape. the small jump on the right occurs during the insertion of the ball, where only residual oil is pushed into the capsule. The pressure remains steady after sealing.

5.5 Component Leakage

Leakage of oil, even minuscule amounts causes immediate change of the strain and stress in the MSD and thus also a change of the pressure measured inside the capsule. Continuous leakage would result in drift of the measured pressure compared to the applied outer pressure. While the pressure difference across the MSD is generally small and only induced by the assembly and temperature cross sensitivity, the difference across the backside sealing and electrical feedthrough is much larger and mostly governed by the momentary blood pressure versus the atmospheric pressure. While leakage through the MSD would only occur until the internal pressure matches the blood pressure, it must not occur to prevent the loss of oil into the bloodstream. The backside sealing and electrical feedthrough are less problematic from a medical point of view, as leaking oil would still remain in the implant body, but critical for the function of the implant. The permanent pressure difference would, in the case of leakage, result in continuous loss of oil, first leading to contact between the MSD and MSD bed and later to the MSD being pressed into the pressure transmission channel. This sequence would be accompanied by severe offset drift, especially in its second stage. Furthermore, significant sensitivity drift is to be expected in the second stage, when the

MSD is heavily deformed and pushed into the pressure transmission channel. This might also affect the blood flow across the MSD and the cavity created by the sunken MSD might give rise to increased blood clotting.

To ensure reliable operation of the capsule concept, each of the three components, MSD, electrical feedthrough, and backside sealing was tested by Helium leak detection, one of the most sensitive techniques available.

The backside sealing was investigated by Pascal Mueller [48], comparing traditional ball-only approaches to the ball-cup solution used in this work, also considering the surface roughness of the cup. He-leak was detectable only in 1/10 ball-only and none of the ball-cup sealings, irrespective of surface roughness.

The electrical feedthrough solder-seal was investigated by Roland Graf [44]. Multiple low temperature solders and a wide parameter range were studied to explore the reliability of the sealing under non-optimal fabrication conditions. Solder sealing was proven to be a highly reliable and robust process.

The nanostructure anchored MSDs, shaped by nanostructure patterning and pressed sugar plug, were investigated by Ian Hutter [43]. The detected He-leak rates matched the calculated expected diffusion rates, indicating that pin-hole free and reliable, damage free manufacturing of MSDs is possible. Additionally, the possibility of oil leaking into the interface between Parylene and nanostructures was investigated and excluded.

6 Implant Characterization

The characteristic properties of MSPSEs are pressure transmission, temperature cross sensitivity and drift (ch. 3.1). This chapter lays out the methods used for characterization and the resulting data from the selected implants. A table with all implants can be found in A.1.

A colored version of this chapter is available at: https://doi.org/10.3929/ethz-b-000702759

6.1 Pressure Transmission

Pressure transmission describes how much of the externally applied pressure is transmitted through the MSD to the sensor inside of the capsule (eq. 3.1). A custom made, voice coil driven, hydrostatic pressure test setup was used for this purpose. The use of static pressure is mandatory to isolate pressure errors caused by the MSD from those caused by fluid dynamic effects under flow.

6.1.1 Materials & Methods

For static pressure measurements, two implants or cannulas were connected to the test station (as described in [40]) and the station was filled with silicone oil (fig. 6.1). Figure A.1 shows the test station with multiple ports occupied by implants without housing. After removing as much air from the system as possible by decreasing and increasing the pressure inside the station, current was applied to the voice coil driving the station's MSD in a stepped pyramidal manner (fig. 6.2) to obtain pressures over a range of more than 26.7 kPa (200 mmHg). For this, the required current in the voice coil to reach a pressure above 26.7 kPa (200 mmHg) was first determined, then a Labview software was used to produce a 10 steps current increase to that value. The reference channel refers to an unencapsulated pressure sensor of the same type as the encapsulated ones directly measuring the pressure inside the tank. The pressure transmission error is calculated as $p_{capsule} - p_{ref} - p_{capsule,0} + p_{ref,0}$. Averaged pressure for each plateau was acquired by step-detection script (Fig. 6.2, the star-marks), excluding a few points around the step.

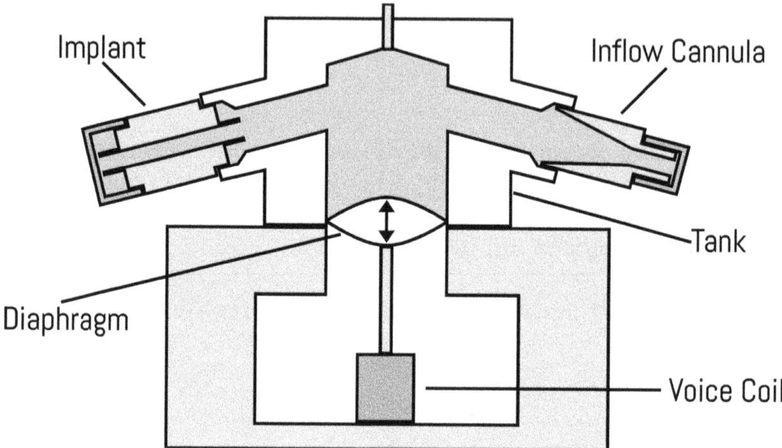

Figure 6.1: Schematic of the cross-section of the pressure transmission testing station. An implant (left) and an inflow cannula (right) are attached to the station. Both are closed on the outer side by a cup (green). The coil drive (orange) at the bottom is used to apply pressure inside the tank via transmission rod and flexible MSD.

6.1.2 Results & Discussion

Figure 6.3 shows the deviation of the recorded pressure by the capsules of the implants from the pressure recorded by the unencapsulated reference sensor versus the pressure recorded by the unencapsulated reference sensor. Capsule 5 of implant 1 and capsule 2 of implant 2 were excluded due to strong hysteresis and the lack of signal, respectively. The deviation over a range of more than 26.7 kPa (200 mmHg) remains within a ± 133 Pa (1 mmHg) window for all displayed capsules. The downward slope, indicating incomplete pressure transmission, is expected as a result of the resistance to deformation of the MSD. Figure 6.4 shows the deviation for all capsules at the highest applied pressure, after off-set calibration to the unencapsulated reference sensor at the lowest applied pressure, divided by the measured pressure range (fig. 6.3, x-axis). The deviation of 0.15 % to 0.3 % would result in a deviation of 40 Pa to 80 Pa (0.3 mmHg to 0.6 mmHg) for the target operating range of 26.7 kPa (200 mmHg).

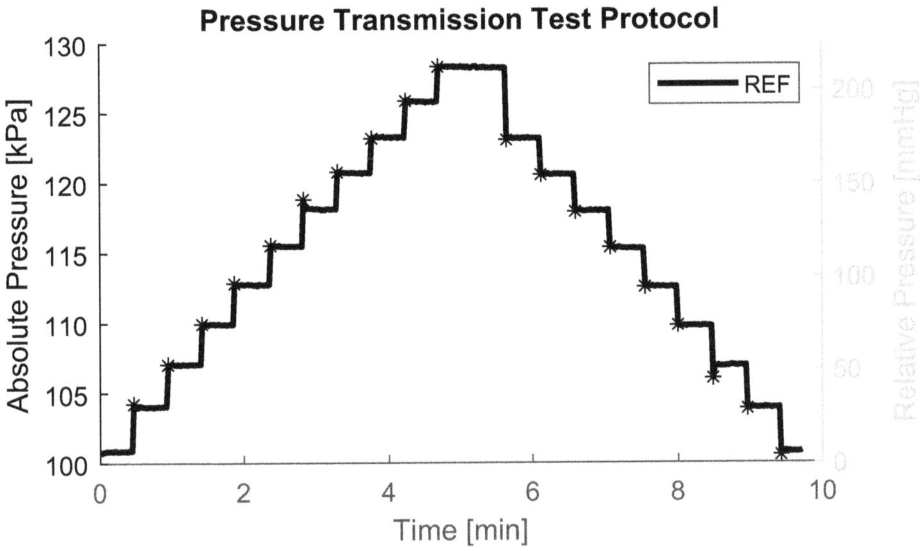

Figure 6.2: Example of the applied pressure profile for pressure transmission testing recorded by the unencapsulated sensor. The asterisks show the automatically detect jumps.

The calculated deviation over a range of 26.7 kPa is 65 Pa (i.e. 0.24% of the range, black line fig. 6.4) for the target MSD thickness of 20 µm and minimal oil-fill pressure of 2 kPa (fig. 3.19). The MSD thickness was measured to be around 19.5 µm to 20 µm on a glass slide placed inside the Parylene coating machine along with implants (as described in ch. 5.1).

Figure 6.5 shows the effect of different minimal pressures during the oil filling process. 3 kPa would already result in a pressure transmission error of 100 Pa. Since the implants were placed in the vacuum chamber and evacuated one by one, it seems reasonable to expect that the lowest achieved pressure during the oil filling process varied across the implants. Additionally, the gentle tapping of the implants during the vacuum step, which helped release air-bubbles (e.g. from the fill channel) could have affected each capsule differently, depending on the position and experienced impact.

It should also be noted that the trueness uncertainty of the sensor (LPS 22) is $\pm$ 10 Pa. For the differential measurement as performed here the uncertainty becomes $\pm$ 20 Pa. Additionally, some variation in Parylene layer thickness can be expected.

Within the confinement of these limitations, the measured pressure transmission is in reasonable agreement with the model.

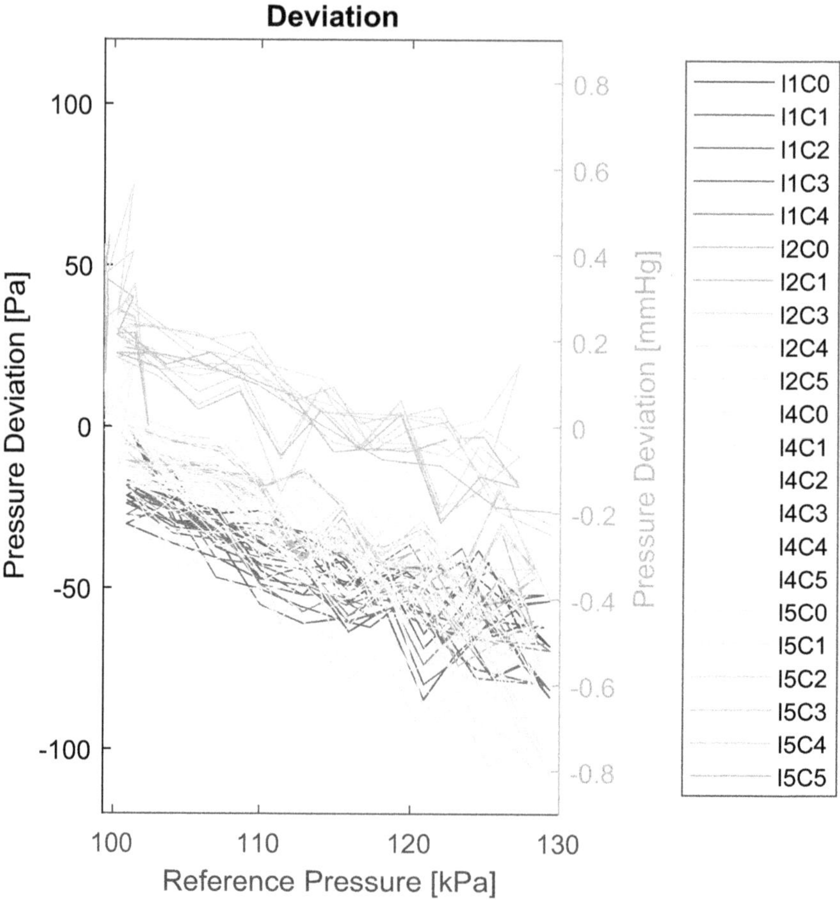

Figure 6.3: Pressure deviation change of the capsules in the implants to the reference sensor. The downward trend indicates reduced pressure transmission for increasing pressures. The pressure transmission error is less than 1 mmHg for all capsules. Two implants were measured per test (I1,I2 then I4,I5). The tested range was slighlty different for the two tests, resulting a difference in tested range for the two batches.

6.1.3 Conclusion

All functioning capsules, with one exception, show excellent pressure transmission with a transmission loss well within the acceptable range. This confirms the encapsulation approach as well as the used model from a pure pressure transmission point of view.

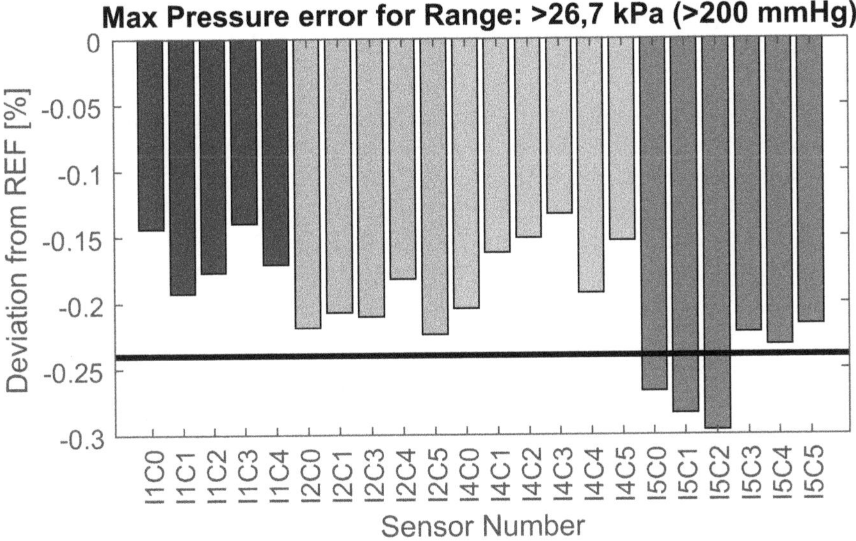

Figure 6.4: Deviation at the highest applied pressure over the measured range, after off-set calibration at the lowest applied pressure. The black line shows the model based, calculated deviation.

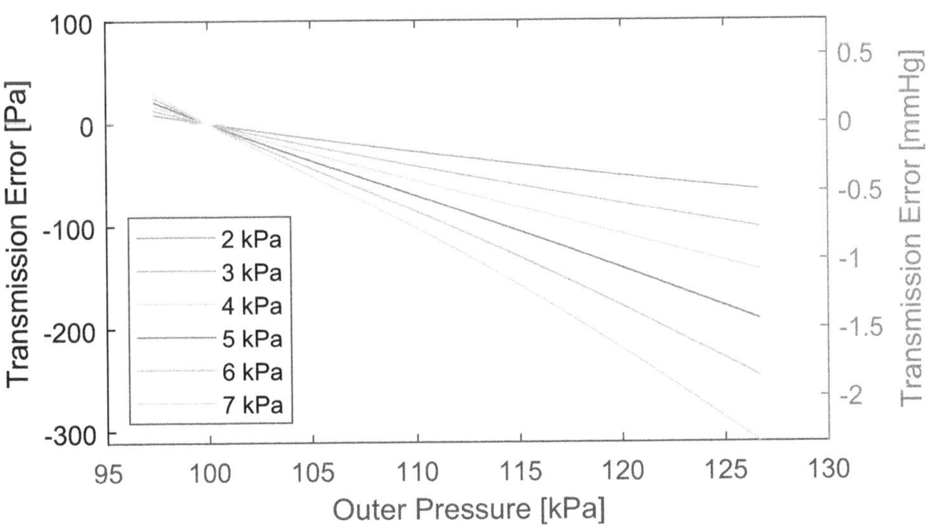

Figure 6.5: Calculated pressure transmission error for a flat pill shaped MSD with r = 1.88 mm, l = 8 mm, h = 20 µm, depending on the lowest achieved pressure during the oil fill process (range: 2 kPa to 7 kPa).

6.2 Temperature Cross Sensitivity

Temperature cross sensitivity (TCS) describes a component of the measured pressure attributed to a change in capsule temperature, which is unrelated to outside pressure changes. In a pressure sensor encapsulation, this can be caused by the difference in CTE between the encapsulated pressure transmission liquid and the surrounding materials (ch. 3.3). This work's silicone oil's CTE is around 40 times larger than that of titanium, in general causing a positive TCS. For the operation of the capsules in-vivo, two values are important. First the TCS around the point of operation. This value should ideally be low enough to guarantee an error within the tolerable range. The second is the pressure increase caused by the heating of the implant to body temperature. This increase in pressure causes an imbalance between the two sides of the MSD, introducing off-set drift into the system (see fig. 3.10) (ch. 3.3). In this section these two aspects of TCS are explored individually. The resulting drift is described in detail in the next chapter.

6.2.1 Materials & Methods

To measure the TCS around the point of operation, the implants were placed in a climate chamber (VCL 4006, Voetsch, Germany) and heated up to body temperature over the course of two hours. Then the chamber was set to oscillate the temperature between 35°C and 42°C using 1 h per cycle (fig. 6.6). Pressure was measured for each capsule by the encapsulated pressure sensor. Temperature was measured by the temperature sensor included in the pressure sensor. TCS coefficients were extracted by automated Matlab script from the oscillating part of the measurement, after subtracting the ambient pressure, measured by an unencapsulated sensor of the same type, placed in the climate chamber along with the implants. The temperature induced pressure error is calculated as $p_{capsule} - p_{ref} - p_{capsule,0} + p_{ref,0}$.

To measure the pressure increase following a temperature change from room to body temperature and its evolution over three cycles, the implants were placed in the above mentioned climate chamber and heated from 23°C to 37°C, where the temperature was maintained for a day, before cooling down again and allowing the implants to rest for a day (fig. 6.7). Pressure was measured for each capsule by the encapsulated pressure sensor. Temperature was measured by the temperature sensor included in the pressure sensor. The pressure difference was measured between a point just before the temperature increase and after the implants reached the upper temperature. Ambient pressure was measured with an unencapsulated sensor of the same type and subtracted from all capsules before evaluation of the pressure measurements.

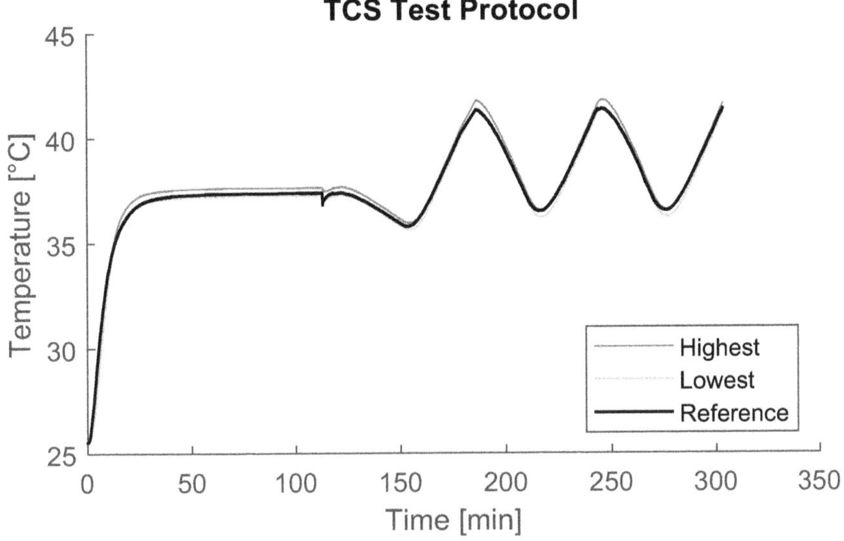

Figure 6.6: TCS measurement protocol, as recorded by the unencapsulated sensor and the capsules with the largest up or down deviation.

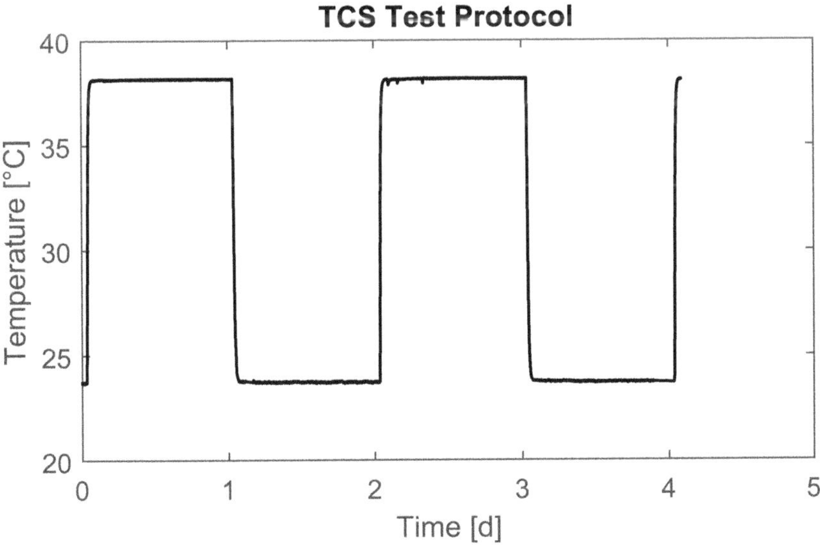

Figure 6.7: TCS measurement protocol for the jump from room to body temperature.

6.2.2 Results & Discussion

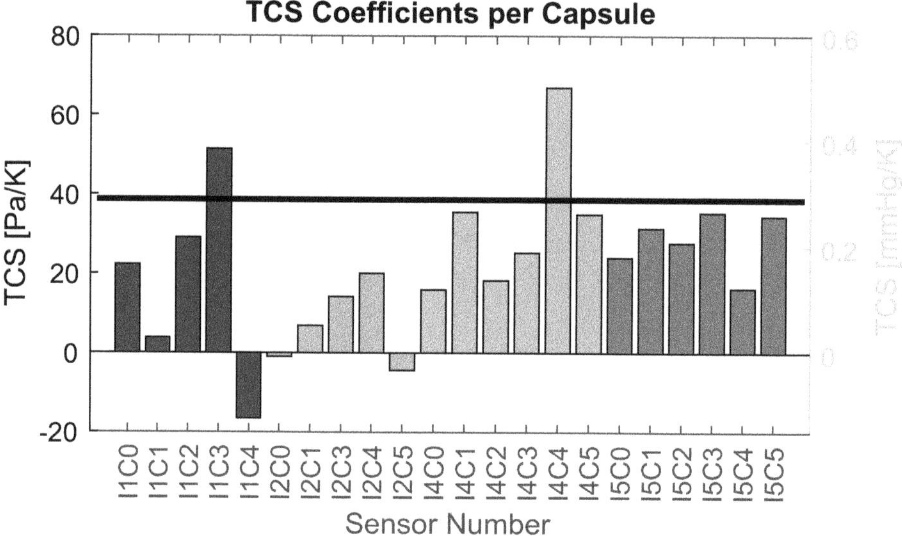

Figure 6.8: TCS coefficients for each capsule around body temperature. The black line shows the 0.29 mmHg/K limit for operation within ±1 mmHg operation from 35°C to 42°C.

Figure 6.6 shows the measured temperature by an un-encapsulated sensor and the highest and lowest measured temperature by the capsules. Some lag can be observed, however, the encapsulation did not suppress the temperature oscillation.

Figure 6.8 shows the measured TCS for each capsule around body temperature. With exception of capsule 3 of the first implant and capsule 4 of implant 4 all TCS coefficients are below the target maximum of 38 Pa (0.29 mmHg/K) (Fig. 6.8, black line). However, a wide variation of TCS coefficients is observable, with some even being negative. Figure 6.9 additionally shows the measured and calculated TCS around body temperature for the cannulae, where incomplete MSD release resulted in a variation of MSD shapes and reduced areas. The values for the MSPSE discussed here, where the MSD were fully released, are agglomerated on the right end of the figure.

Figure 6.10 shows the pressure increase accompanying the temperature increase from room to body temperature. The increase in pressure is significantly larger than predicted by the model (fig. 3.18). Similarities to the TCS around body temperature can be seen (compare to fig. 6.8) however

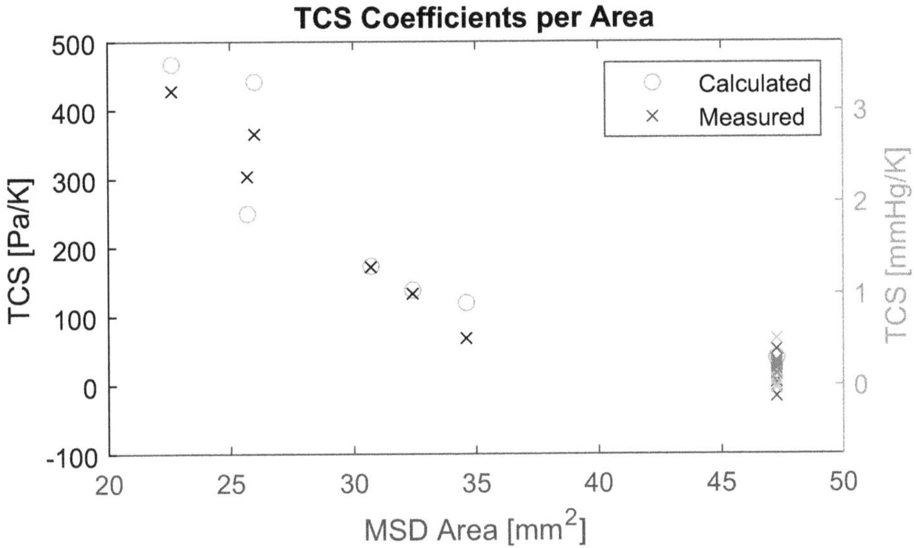

Figure 6.9: Calculated and measured TCS coefficients for the implants (bottom right corner, see fig. 6.8 for details) and for the cannula (from: [46]) around body temperature.

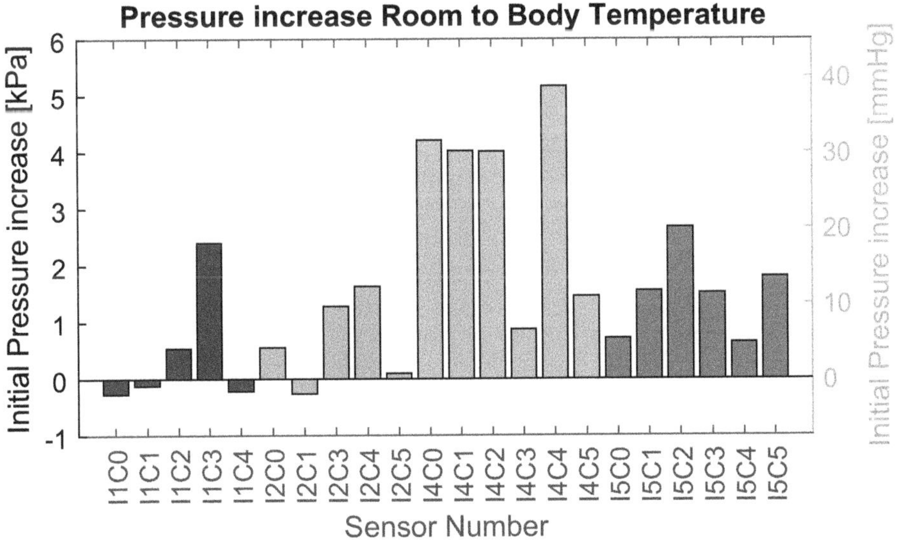

Figure 6.10: Measured pressure increase following a temperature jump from room to body temperature for each capsule. (First jump in fig. 6.7)

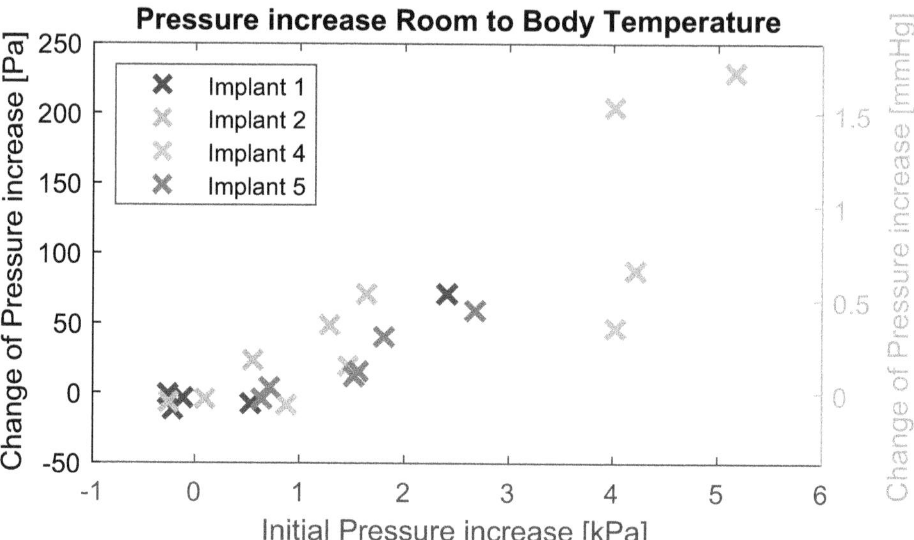

Figure 6.11: Shows the change in pressure increase on the third cycle, 4 days after the first (see: 6.7).

no precise correlation can be observed, indicating that the underlying cause is partially related, but not the same. Furthermore figure 6.11 shows the change of the pressure jump between the first and last temperature increase (fig. 6.7). A wide range of change and a loose correlation between the magnitude of the pressure increase and the change can be observed.

While the model produces a good maximum estimation of the TCS around body temperature, also for MSD of different shapes and overall areas, it severely underestimates the initial pressure increase from room temperature to body temperature. A potential explanation for this could be found in the curvature of the MSD. In its initial state the MSD is in a bridge-arch-like state against the pressure transmission channel and needs to buckle to make room for the expanding pressure transmission fluid. The initial pressure increase could reflect the pressure required for this state transition. The wide range of coefficients could then be caused by different overfilling levels of the capsules after the final sealing step resulting in differently prebuckling of the MSDs.

6.2.3 Conclusion

All functioning capsules with two exceptions showed low enough TCS to not exceed a 266 Pa (2 mmHg) band during operation. The used model served well as a safe estimation for MSD design with respect to the temperature window during operation. However, the temperature increase from room to body temperature resulted in a larger than predicted pressure increase.

6.3 Drift

Drift describes the change of offset (offset drift) or correlation between the outer pressure and the measured pressure (sensitivity drift). In this work the main contributor to drift is the relaxation of the polymer MSD after the pressure increase (offset) caused by the temperature increase from room to body temperature. This relaxation results in a decay of the pressure increase and therefore offset drift.

6.3.1 Materials & Methods

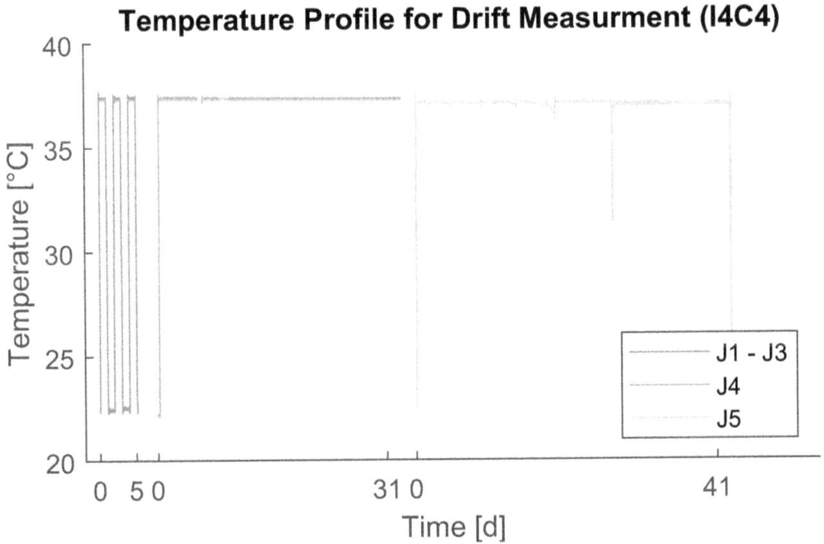

Figure 6.12: Drift measurement protocol to observe temperature induced pressure drift. Temperature as recorded by capsule 4 of implant 4 (I4C4). After increasing the temperature from room to body temperature. the first 3 runs consist of an increase to body temperature followed by a 1 day holding phase before cooling back to room temperature. The 4th and 5th run had a holding time of 33 and 42 days.

To measure drift, the implants were placed in a climate chamber (VCL 4006, Voetsch, Germany) and heated up to body temperature 5 times, where they were left for 1, 1, 1, 33, and 42 days (fig. 6.12). The implants were stored at body temperature for more than a month and cooled to room temperature 1 day before the first test. In-between the first 3 measurments, they were stored at room temperature for 1 day each and for more than 1 week before the 4th and 5th test. When required the climate chamber door was only opened for a minimum amount of time to keep temperature fluctuations minimal. Pressure was measured for each capsule by the encapsulated pressure sensor. Temperature was measured by the temperature sensor included in the pressure sensor. Drift was extracted by automated Matlab script from the isothermal part of the measurement, after subtracting the ambient pressure, measured by an un-encapsulated sensor of the same type, placed in the climate chamber along with the implants. The drift induced error is calculated as $p_{capsule} - p_{ref} - p_{capsule,0} + p_{ref,0}$. I1C3 and I2C4 stopped returning a stable signal and were therefore excluded from this chapter.

6.3.2 Results & Discussion

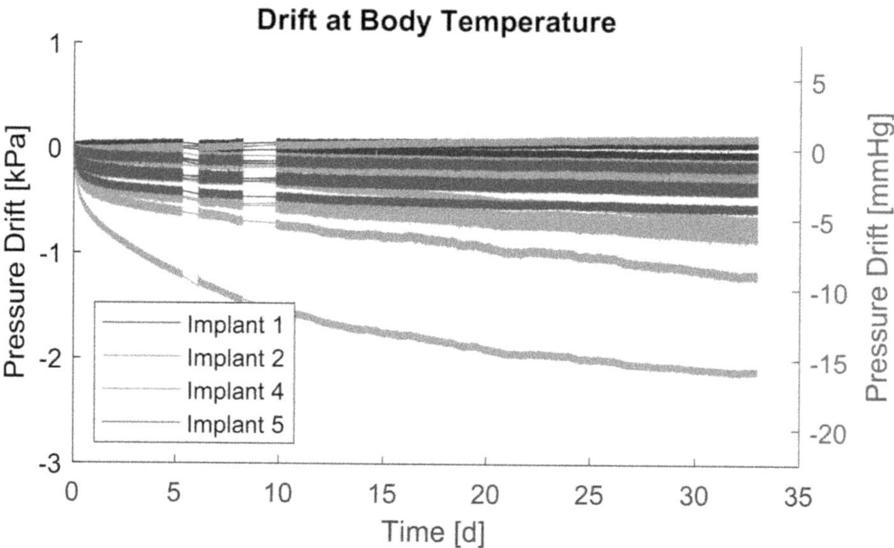

Figure 6.13: Pressure drift after temperature jump 4 over the course of 33 days. (4th run in fig. 6.12, J4; for the other runs see: fig. A.2, A.3, A.4, A.5)

Figure 6.13 shows the pressure drift after reaching body temperature of the 4th run. A strong initial drift phase in the first day can be observed which rapidly decays and stabilizes for most sensors. Figure 6.14 shows the

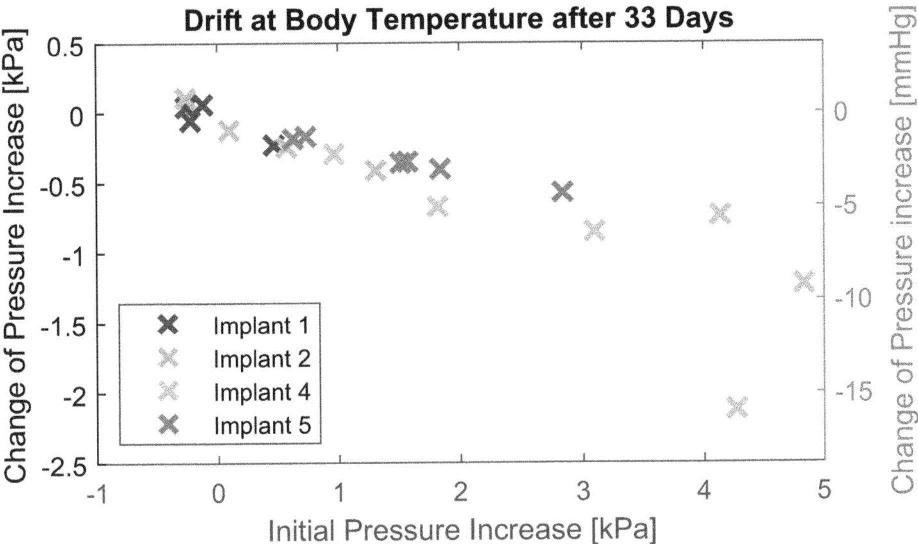

Figure 6.14: Change or thermally induced pressure increase after 33 days in relation to the initial increase. All capsules with one exception follow a similar correlation between initial pressure increase and change of pressure increase over time. (for the other runs see: fig. A.6, A.7, A.8, A.9)

initial temperature induced pressure increase during the temperature jump from room to body temperature (vertical lines in fig. 6.12) and the following measured total pressure offset drift at the end of the experiment (end points of the curves in fig. 6.13, measured from after the jump, to the end of the recorded period). A clear correlation between the two is visible. This is expected as the increased pressure causes more stress in and therefore faster relaxation of the MSD. Figure 6.15 shows the iterative progression of the measured drift of the MSPSEs within the first day and for every period of 10 days afterwards where available as well as the overall drift for all 5 runs. The rapid decay of the drift after the first day is visible for both long term runs.

The first 3 runs show less drift on the first day than runs 4 and 5. This could have been caused by the extended storage of the implants at body temperature, with only one day at room-temperature before and in between the runs. Before runs 4 and 5, the implants were stored at room temperature before the experiment for at least one week. This behaviour matches the expectations for a viscoelastic MSD, where recovery after relaxation progresses slowly with time.

The median drift in the last 10 days of run 4 and 5 is -30 Pa (-0.22 mmHg)

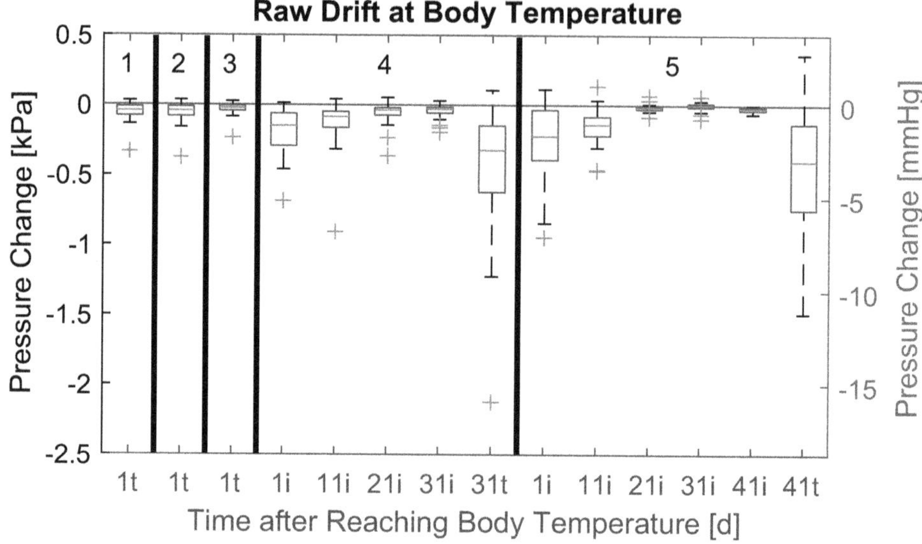

Figure 6.15: Change or thermally induced pressure increase within the first day and following intervals of 10 d (i) and the total drift (t) of all MSPSEs

and -20 Pa (-0.15 mmHg) respectively, which is still higher than the 7 Pa/10 d (0.0548 mmHg/10 d) which results in 2 mmHg/y if linearly extrapolated.

6.3.3 Conclusion

All functioning capsules with one exception showed a similar drift pattern and the expected correlation between initial pressure increase and drift was observed clearly. The temperature induced drift was found to rapidly decay within the first 11 days but to remain 3-4 time larger than the desired target value. However, the found correlation might offer a path towards error correction.

7 Error Reduction for Implants

This chapter discusses the possibility to reduce various types of deviations of the measured intra-capsular pressure from the outer pressure. Specifically a linear correction of the pressure transmission based on calibration measurement and a differential sensing method used to correct temperature induced effects. The later is based on the scaling of drift with the initial pressure increase observed in the previous chapter. The methods explored in this chapter are based solely on pressure measurements and do not rely on temperature or time, with the exception that compared measurements need to be taken at the same time.

A colored version of this chapter is available at: https://doi.org/10.3929/ethz-b-000702759

7.1 Pressure Transmission Correction

While the pressure transmission error was found to be low and matching with the expected values (ch. 6.1), further reduction can contribute to a reduced total error.

7.1.1 Materials & Methods

A linear correction based on the individual difference between the unencapsulated sensor and each capsule at the highest and lowest measured pressures was used (see eq. 7.1). The residual error after correction for all measured pressures is described here. Noise was not considered, as the measured pressures are averaged across a step (see fig. 6.2).

$$p_{p-corr}(t) = (p(t) - p_{min})\frac{p_{c,max} - p_{c,min}}{p_{max} - p_{min}} + p_{c,min} \tag{7.1}$$

where $p_{p-corr}(t)$ is the pressure transmission corrected pressure, $p(t)$ is the pressure measured by the encapsulated sensor, p_{min} and p_{max} are the linearly fitted pressures measured by the encapsulated sensor during the calibration at the lowest and highest applied pressures, and $p_{c,min}$ and $p_{c,max}$ are the lowest and highest pressures measured by an unencapsulated sensor during the calibration. This calibration is performed for each sensor individually, based on its own deviation from the reference sensor.

7.1.2 Results & Discussion

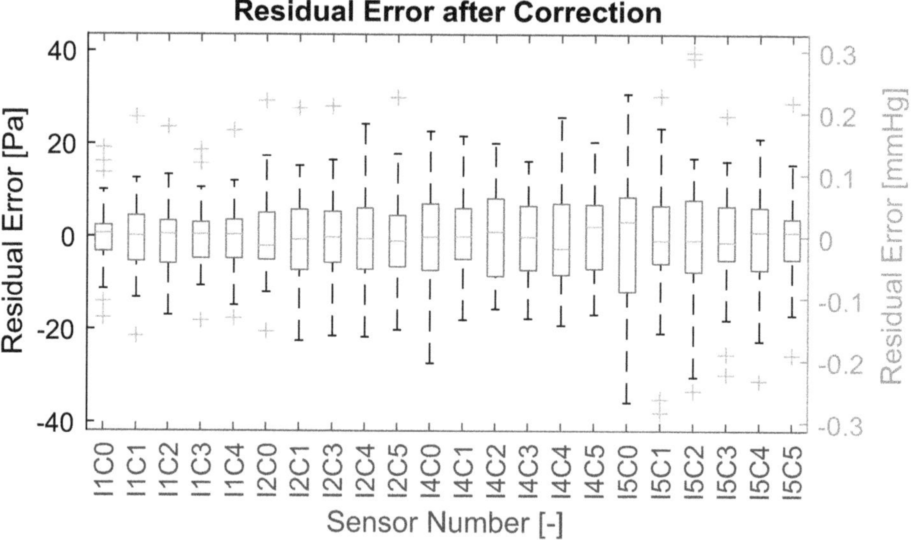

Figure 7.1: Residual pressure transmission error after linear correction. Correction applied to data shown in fig. 6.3.

Figure 7.1 shows the residual error for all measured pressures for each capsule. The correction results in a reduction of the error to 0±10 Pa (0±0.07 mmHg, STD) with all data points within a ±40 Pa (±0.3 mmHg) window. This step reduces the pressure transmission error by up to 50 % or 40 Pa (0.3 mmHg).

7.1.3 Conclusion

Applying a linear correction the pressure transmission can reduce the pressure transmission error and contribute to a smaller total error. Potential pressure transmission sensitivity drift was not further investigated. Pressure offset drift is discussed in the next section.

7.2 Drift Correction

The significant, temperature induced offset drift observed in ch. 6.3 exceeds tolerable error boundaries. However, the scaling of drift with the initial temperature induced pressure increase, as it occurs during implantation, offers a path towards correction. In a practical application, an identically built MSPSE included in the implant, which is not measuring the blood pressure, but a known pressure instead and is thermally connected to the other MSPSEs, could be used to produce a reference drift signal. A schematic of such an assembly is shown in figure 7.2. The enclosed diaphragm separates the incompressible pressure transmission oil from the air compartment. The compressible air side allows the diaphragm to deflect when the oil expands under the influence of temperature. The temperature induced pressure error and drift can be calculated as the difference between the pressures on both sides and the air pressure can either be calculated via ideal gas law and recorded temperature or by a second pressure sensor.

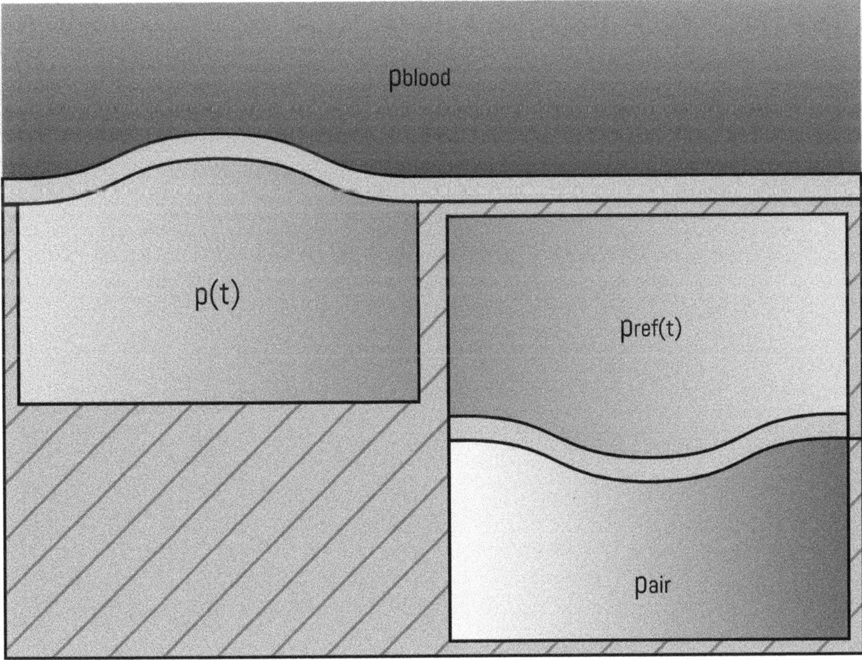

Figure 7.2: Schematic of a reference capsule. The reference sensor is placed inside the oil side. A second sensor could also placed in the air side to remove pressure uncertainty on the gas side.

With such a reference signal the drift correction could be executed following:

$$p_{d-corr}(t) = p(t) - \Delta p_{ref,th}(t) \frac{\Delta p_{th}}{\Delta p_{ref,th}} \tag{7.2}$$

where $p_{d-corr}(t)$ is the drift corrected pressure, $p(t)$ is the pressure measured by the encapsulated sensor, $\Delta p_{ref,th}(t)$ is the pressure measured by second, identically encapsulated sensor measuring a known pressure minus the pressure it measured before the temperature jump, and Δp_{th} and $\Delta p_{ref,th}$ are the thermally induced pressure increases from room to body temperature. (t) indicates that measurements need to be taken at the same time. Here such a sensor is simulated by using the median of the drift curves normalized to their initial pressure increase, of all capsules per implant and it's drift is referred to as the characteristic drift profile. This was done implant-wise as it is assumed, that all capsules on one implant share a very similar thermal history, which was observed to affect the drift pattern in ch. 6.3.

In a scenario where two blood pressure measuring MSPSE and no reference MSPSE are available eq. 7.2 can be transformed (in detail, see sec. A.2) to:

$$p_{1,d-corr}(t) = \frac{p_1(t) * \Delta p_{2,th} - p_2(t) * \Delta p_{1,th}}{\Delta p_{2,th} - \Delta p_{1,th}} \tag{7.3}$$

Where the index 1 and 2 describe values assigned to the first and second MSPSE.

A model based correction approach is described in chapter 8.

7.2.1 Materials & Methods

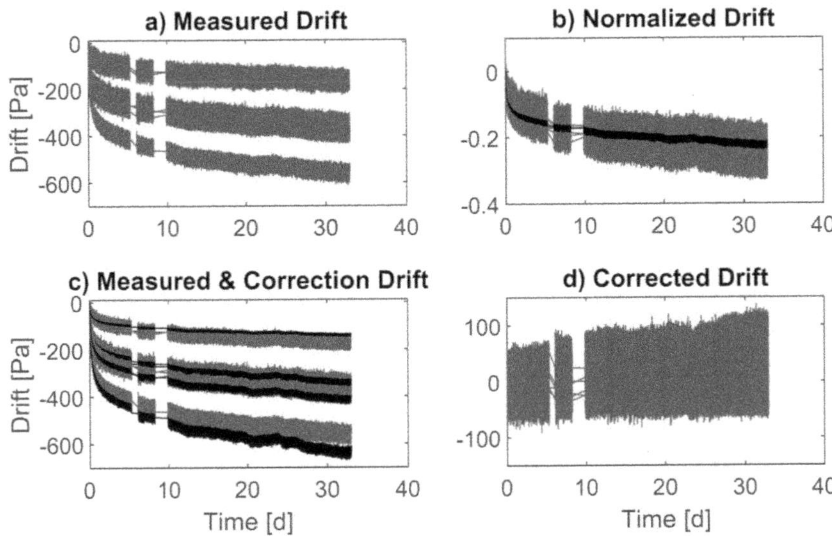

Figure 7.3: Process flow of the drift correction process. Example data of implant 5, from run 4 is shown here. a) The drift as measured. b) drift normalized by the initial pressure jump (red) and the median normalized drift (black). c) the measured drift (red) and the median normalized drift multiplied by the individual initial jump (black). d) residual drift error after drift correction.

For each implant and each run a characteristic drift profile was extracted as the median of the pressure drift of each capsule divided by it's initial pressure increase (Fig.7.3 b). The characteristic drift profile was then multiplied by the initial pressure increase (i.e. pressure increase during the temperature jump from room to body temperature, see fig. 6.14) of each capsule (Fig.7.3 c) and subtracted from the measured drift (Fig.7.3 d). I1C3 and I2C4 stopped returning a stable signal and were therefore excluded from this chapter. This calibration is performed for each run, for each sensor individually, based on its own initial pressure increase and the normalized median drift of all sensors on the same implant.

7.2.2 Results & Discussion

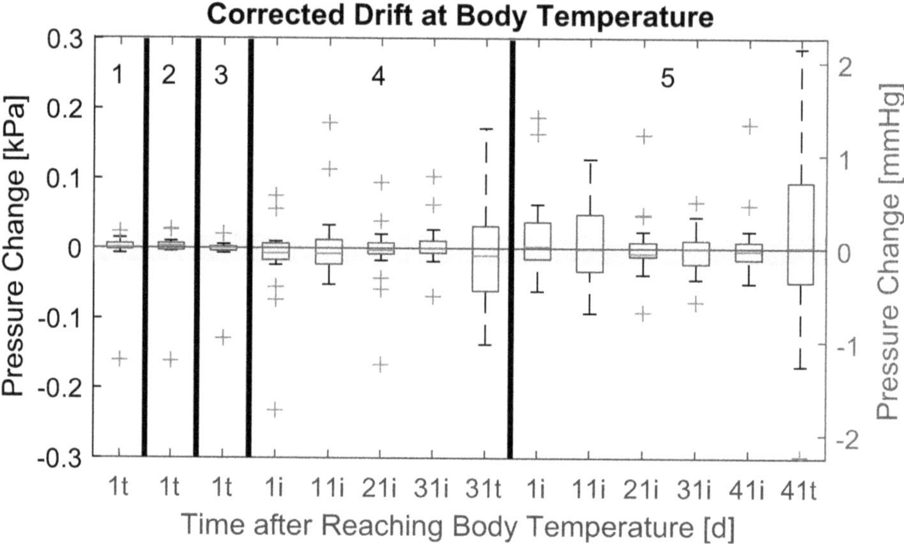

Figure 7.4: Residual error after implant- and run wise drift correction. For the first day, then for intervals of 10 d and the total duration. The orange area shows the sensor's uncertainty range. All outliers visible in fig. A.10.

Figure 7.3 shows the scaling of the drift profile with the initial pressure increase. The as-measured pressure decay profiles (fig. 7.3, a) collapse into a single curve (fig. 7.3, b) after division by their individual initial pressure increases. In reverse, the median normalized drift profile, multiplied by the individual initial pressure increase, also matches the as-measured drift profiles well (fig. 7.3, c). The residual error after correction (the difference between the two), therefore becomes small. The residual error seen here is attributed to variations in the manufacturing process.

Figure 7.4 shows the residual error after drift correction and shows the significant error reduction both for the iterative drift error as well as the overall error (compare to fig. 6.15). The two total median residual error values and all decadal, except the first of run 4 (-7.5 Pa or -0.056 mmHg) are within the permissive limits (7.3 Pa per 10 days corresponding to 2 mmHg/y).

The narrowest residual day 1 error distribution can be found for the first 3 runs. This could indicate that storing the capsules at body temperature would significantly reduce drift variations upon implantation, even if the they are exposed to room temperature for 24 h in-between. The lower and

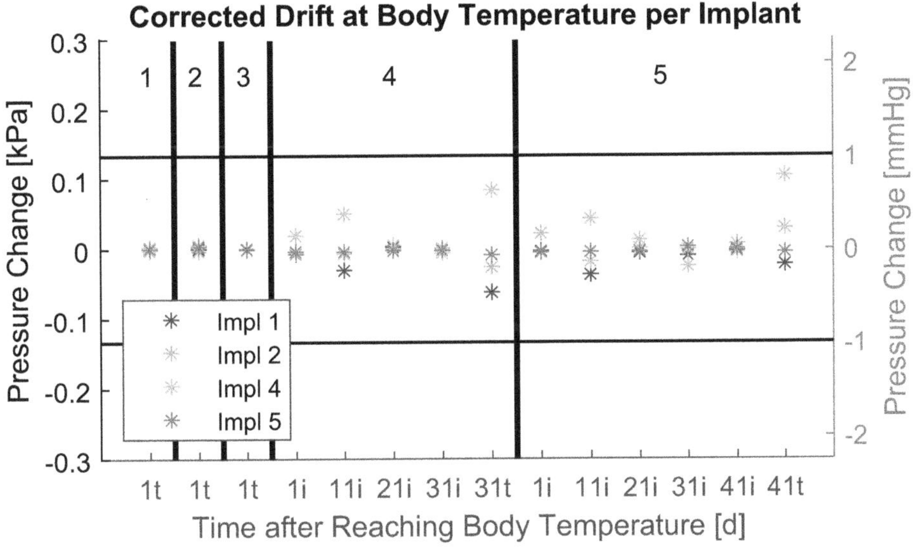

Figure 7.5: Residual error after implant-wise averaging and omission of the least agreeing sensor per implant.

upper quartiles of the decadal errors remain within -32 Pa (-0.24 mmHg) and 50 Pa (0.37 mmHg), which corresponds to the quartiles of the first decade of the 5 runs. All other nearly fit within the uncertainty band of the sensor itself (orange band fig. 7.4). The overall residual error quartiles for run 4 and 5 are -61 Pa (-0.46 mmHg) to 32 Pa 0.24 mmHg and -48 Pa (-0.36 mmHg) to 95 Pa (0.71 mmHg) respectively. Assuming the residual error in the last decade of run 4 and 5 remains steady after the total error measurement, the extrapolated annual drift for each capsule leaves 5, 8, and 12 out of 20 within an annual drift window of ±133 Pa (±1 mmHg), ±266 Pa (±2 mmHg), and ±399 Pa (±3 mmHg) for run 4 and 4, 6, and 9 out of 20 within the same windows for run 5.

Here a reference sensor was emulated by using the median of the normalized drift profiles. In an application scenario, the reference sensor would be subject to the same distribution as the measuring sensors, potentially perfectly eliminating but also potentially doubling residual error.

Considering each implant as a sensor system offers additional information on the behaviour of the capsules in operation such as clustering and potential outlier detection. For the 4 implants discussed in this work, the residual error can be further reduced by omitting the capsule furthest from their mean value and averaging the pressure over the remaining capsules. Figure 7.5 shows this for each implant, leaving the residual error within

±133 Pa (±1 mmHg) for all scenarios. Extrapolation to annual residual errors leaves all implants for both projections, based on run 4 and 5 within the ±133 Pa (±1 mmHg) window, with exception of Implant 2 with run 5 which results in 333 Pa (2.5 mmHg) (fig. A.11).

7.2.3 Conclusion

The described drift correction method significantly reduces the drift error per capsule especially in the initial phase after a temperature jump. This shows that the most significant component of pressure drift is caused by thermal cross sensitivity and that the drift follows a very similar profile for all capsules. The remaining residual error can be reduced by exploiting the multiple capsules built into each implant.

7.3 Temperature Cross Sensitivity Correction

The temperature cross sensitivity around body temperature as described in chapter (ch. 6.2) will naturally be affected by the drift correction method. Since the drift correction method is based on the scaling between two signals with the initial pressure increase and small temperature induced pressure fluctuations scale very similarly with the large initial pressure increase (fig. 6.11), a positive effect on the TCS coefficients after correction is to be expected.

7.3.1 Materials & Methods

The same experimental data described in chapter (ch. 6.2) was used and processed as described above (ch. 7.2).

7.3.2 Results & Discussion

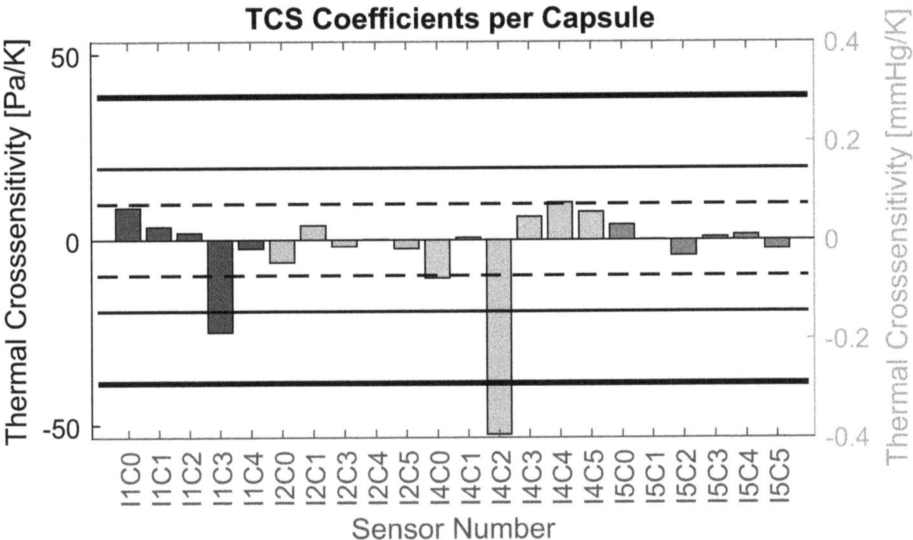

Figure 7.6: TCS after drift correction. The drift correction method also reduces the TCS for most MSPSE. Uncorrected TCS from the same test visible in fig. 6.8.

Figure 7.6 shows the extracted TCS coefficients after correction (data from fig. 6.8, corrected as in fig. 7.3). The thick lines show the design target range for 266 Pa (±2 mmHg) operation in a window from 35°C to 42°C. The fine line depicts the 133 Pa (±1 mmHg) and the dashed line the 67 Pa (±0.5 mmHg) range. With 2 exceptions, all capsules are at, or inside the later. Only one TCS coefficient remains outside the target window. However, its magnitude is less then the largest in the uncorrected evaluation.

These results show that the local TCS coefficients scale to some extent with the initial pressure jumps while heating the implants from room to body temperature. This is not surprising, as they are in essence a continuation of the initial jumps. It can therefore be assumed, that they will change over time as the initial jumps do (fig. 6.11) and should therefore remain corrected with the described correction method. However, some residual error remains, which is attributed to the variation in individual scaling observed in ch. 6.2.

7.3.3 Conclusion

The described drift correction method also significantly reduces the local TCS around the point of operation, strongly reducing the need for additional temperature correction in the operation temperature window.

7.4 Overall Residual Error

Three sources of uncertainty have been considered and corrected, pressure transmission (ch. 7.1), temperature cross sensitivity around body temperature (ch. 7.3), and temperature induced drift (ch. 7.2). Figure 7.7 shows a superposition of the residual drift error at 41 d of run 5 and the residual uncertainty window for pressure transmission (as the largest positive and negative value) and TCS (from 35°C to 42°C as TCS coefficient multiplied by 5°C and -2°C) after correction for each capsule. The drift error compared to the error ranges of the other two sources can be seen side by side in figure 7.8. While none of the three error sources dominates over the others for all sensors, it can be seen the drift causes the largest errors and is most frequently the most significant contributor. Additionally, it must be considered that the drift error, also after correction, will continuously increase over time. Projections for 3 months based on the total drift at day 41 and the mean decadal drift of the last two decades of the 4th and 5th drift experiment can be found in the appendix (fig. A.12, fig A.13 and fig. A.14, fig A.15). Table 7.1 shows how many sensors remain fully within (+), are at the border of (o) or outside (-) of a ±3 mmHg window.

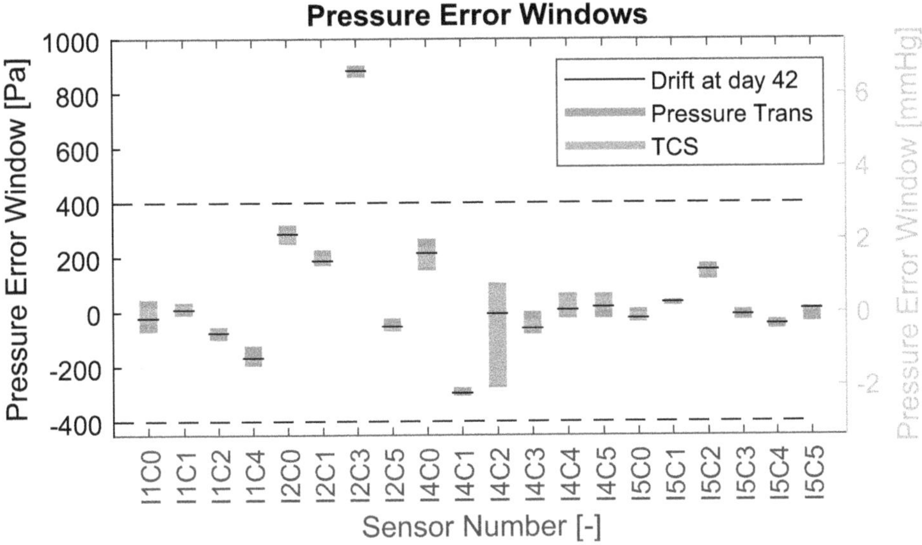

Figure 7.7: The error window after correction as a combination of the measured drift error, combined with the error windows for pressure and TCS, for each sensor individually. The dashed line represents a ±3 mmHg window.

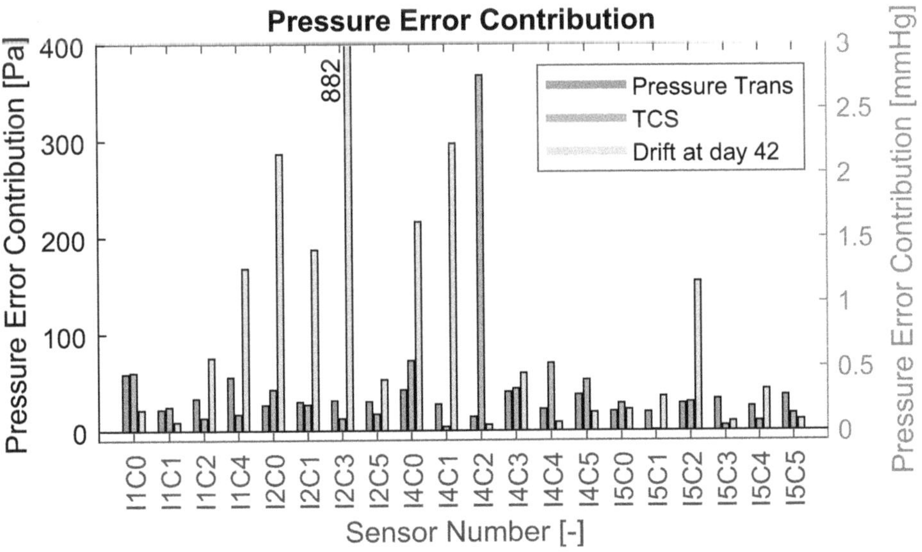

Figure 7.8: Residual error sources after correction next to each other.

Table 7.1: Classification of the capsules based on the fulfilment of the ±3 mmHg maximal error window for the combined measurement errors (41 d) and with drift projections for 3 months and 1 year. A + denotes capsules within, a o capsules on the border of and a - capsules outside of the target window. I1C3 and I2C4 stopped returning a stable signal and were therefore excluded from this chapter.

Capsules	41 days	3 months	1 year
I1 C0	+	+	+
I1 C1	+	+	+
I1 C2	+	+	+
I1 C4	+	+	-
I2 C0	o	o	-
I2 C1	+	o	-
I2 C3	-	-	-
I2 C5	+	+	+
I4 C0	o	o	-
I4 C1	+	+	-
I4 C2	+	+	o
I4 C3	+	+	+
I4 C4	+	+	-
I4 C5	+	+	-
I5 C0	+	+	+
I5 C1	+	+	+
I5 C2	+	+	-
I5 C3	+	+	+
I5 C4	+	+	+
I5 C5	+	+	+

While not part of the encapsulation, additionally, the single sensor noise itself has to be considered and is 6.5 Pa RMS.

7.4.1 Suggested approach

For the pressure correction, an in-vitro measurement to acquire the pressure transmission error is required. For the TCS and Drift correction a second, identical capsule is required. This second capsule must be implemented near the main capsule to experience the same thermal history and measure a known pressure. Additionally a pressure measurement during the implantation of the device is required. With these components, the pressure correction can be executed as follows

$$p_{corr}(t) = (p(t) - p_{ref}(t)\frac{\Delta p_{th}}{\Delta p_{ref,th}}) - p_{min})\frac{p_{c,max} - p_{c,min}}{p_{max} - p_{min}} + p_{c,min} \quad (7.4)$$

where $p_{corr}(t)$ is the corrected pressure, $p(t)$ is the pressure measured by the encapsulated sensor, $p_{ref}(t)$ is the pressure measured by second, identically encapsulated sensor, and Δp_{th} and $\Delta p_{ref,th}$ are the thermally induced pressure increases from room to body temperature. Note that the drift correction must be corrected before the pressure transmission error to avoid wrongfully scaling the drift error, unless pressure transmission was already corrected during the acquisition of the pressure measurement during implantation.

8 Model Based TCS Correction

A colored version of this chapter is available at: https://doi.org/10.3929/ethz-b-000702759

8.1 Burgers Model Based Correction

Temperature cross sensitivity is the most significant component of the total error of the described implants. Temperature cross sensitivity is introduced by the CTE mismatch between the different components of the MSPSEs and contains a time dependent component originating from the viscoelastic MSD material. This time dependent component is especially pronounced immediately after a temperature change which occurs during the implantation. The Burgers model (fig. 8.1) is employed here to predict the temperature induced pressure error based solely on the temperature recording of the integrated temperature sensor and a starting state. The model used here equates

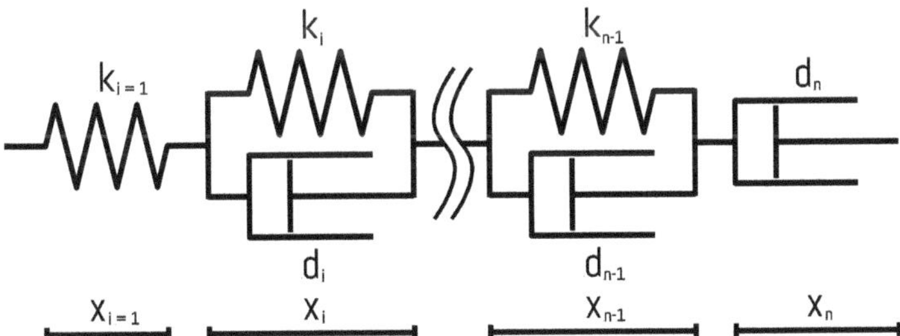

Figure 8.1: Schematic of the Burgers Model as it is used in this chapter. The spring on the left side and the dampener on the right side are always present. The number of combined spring/dampener elements can vary. Here a model with one (1/1/1) and two (1/2/1) such elements is used.

the stretching of the MSD by the expansion of the pressure transmission oil with the stretching of the burgers model's element chain. The temperature induced pressure increase is equated with the force of the Burgers model. The total length of all elements (corresponding to the temperature) is:

$$T_{lin}(t) \cong X(t)\frac{K}{m} = \sum_{1}^{n} x_i(t)\frac{K}{m} \tag{8.1}$$

where:

- $T_{lin}(t)$ is the "linearized" temperature (see fig. 8.2)
- t is the time
- $X(t)$ is the total length of the Burgers model chain
- $x_i(t)$ is the length of element i

and the force (corresponding to the pressure) is:

$$p_{Calc}(t) \cong F(t)\frac{Pa}{N} = k_i x_i(t)\frac{Pa}{N} + d_i\frac{\partial x_i(t)}{\partial t}\frac{Pa}{N} \tag{8.2}$$

where:

- $p_{Calc}(t)$ is the predicted pressure
- $F(t)$ is the force across the Burgers chain
- k_i is the spring constant of element i
- d_i is the dampening constant if element i

and is implemented as a step from t_j to t_{j+1} as:

$$p_{Calc}(t_{j+1}) \cong F(t_{j+1})\frac{Pa}{N} = k_i x_i(t_{j+1})\frac{Pa}{N} + d_i\frac{x_i(t_{j+1}) - x_i(t_j)}{t_{j+1} - t_j}\frac{Pa}{N} \tag{8.3}$$

where:

- t_j is the element j of the discreet time recording
- t_{j+1} is the element j+1 of the discreet time recording

It should be noted that eq. 8.3 becomes independent of the previous point in time for the pure spring element $d_1 = 0$, as the pure spring element is assumed to react instantaneously.

Replacing each element length $x_i(t_{j+1})$ in eq. 8.1 at t_{j+1} by eq. 8.3 results in (in detail, see sec. A.3):

$$p_{Calc}(t_{j+1}) = \frac{T_{lin}(t_{j+1}) - \sum_1^n \frac{d_i \frac{x_i}{t_{j+1}-t_i}}{k_i + \frac{d_i}{t_{j+1}-t_j}}}{\sum_1^n \frac{1}{k_i + d_i/(t_{j+1}-t_j)}} \frac{Pa}{N} \tag{8.4}$$

The system wise units of each variable are shown in table 8.1.

Table 8.1: Side by side comparison of the variables used to describe the MSPSEs temperature induced error with their units for both systems.

p(T) system	Units	Burgers Model	Units
T	K	X	m
p	Pa	F	N
t	s	t	s
k	Pa/K	k	N/m
d	Pas/K	d	Ns/m

Additionally, the non-linear relationship between the measured temperature and stretching of the MSD is quasi-linearized by cubic polynomial transformation first. The parameter for the cubic function are extracted by fitting to four points taken on a slow step profile ramp and used to convert the recorded temperature (fig. 8.2) using:

$$T_{lin}(t) = a * (T_{Meas}(t))^3 + b * (T_{Meas}(t))^2 + c * T_{Meas}(t) + d \tag{8.5}$$

where:

- $T_{lin}(t)$ is the "linearized" temperature
- $T_{Meas}(t)$ is the measured temperature
- a, b, c, d are the parameter of the cubic equation

8.1.1 Materials & Methods

After an initial manual first guess fit, all parameter sets were passed to the optimization algorithm. For each optimization cycle (fig. 8.3), parameter variation of the fitting parameter $\vec{k}$, $\vec{d}$ and the pressure offset were prepared, creating a slightly increased and slightly decreased variation. The cubic parameter set a, b, c, d was left unchanged.

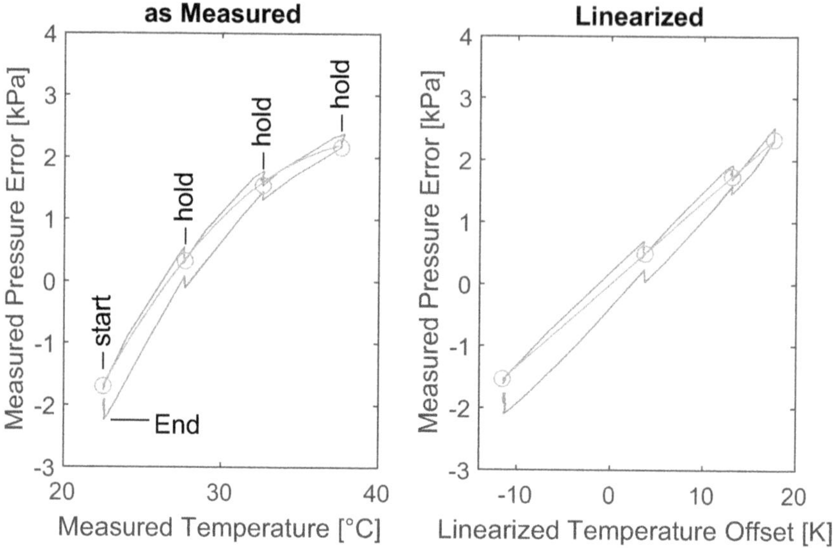

Figure 8.2: Left: The measured pressure and temperature, the fitted function and the points used for fitting. A stepped temperature profile was used to enable all MSPSE to stabilize at each temperature point and reduce the influence of the high drift rates immediately after the temperature jumps. Right: The linearized relation.

In a first step, the pressure-temperature relation is "linearized" by transforming the temperature measurement using the cubic function (eq. 8.5). Then, for every calculation, as a starting condition it is assumed that all spring components exert the same force (i.e. that the model reached a steady state) using:

$$\vec{x}(t_1) = p_{Meas}(t_1)/\vec{k} \tag{8.6}$$

where:

- $\vec{x}$ is the element length vector $(x_1, x_2, ...x_n)$
- $\vec{k}$ is the spring constant vector $(k_1, k_2, ...k_n)$
- $p_{Meas}(t_1)$ is the first measured pressure

To match this as closely as possible, the fitting was done for a part of the recorded data starting after a prolonged exposure of the implants to constant temperature. Then the pressure was iteratively calculated for each measured

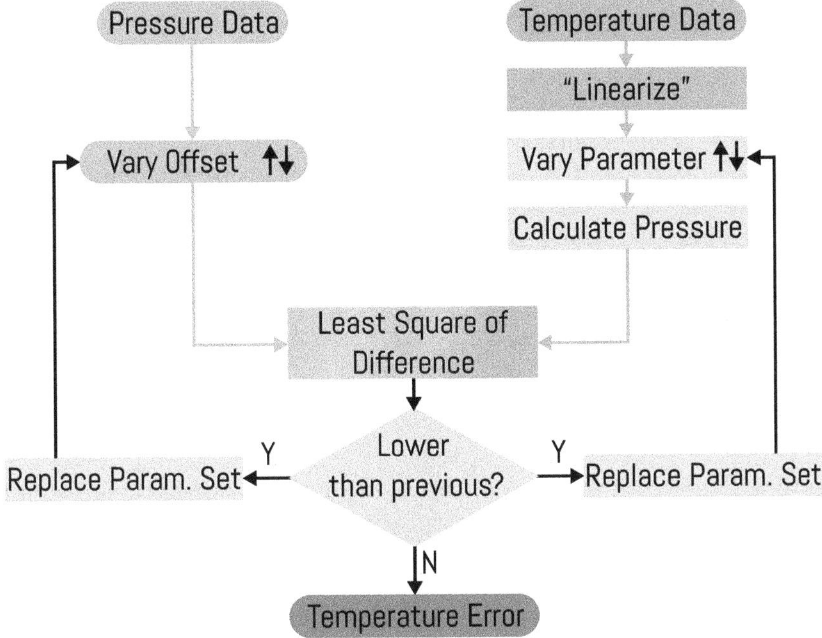

Figure 8.3: The flowchart represents the Burgers model parameter fitting process. On the left side the measured pressure data offset is varied, which governs the initial length of the Burgers model element chain. On the right side the temperature data is adjusted to create a more linear pressure to temperature relation. Then all the Burgers parameter are varied and the pressure is calculated. The least squares of the difference between the calculated and measured pressures are then evaluated and and the best fitting parameter set is chosen for the next cycle.

point in time using eq. 8.4. This process is repeated for all combinations of all variations.

The parameters leading to the solution with the lowest least squares of the difference of $p_{Meas} - p_{Calc}$ were chosen and the cycle was restarted until the unvaried parameter set was found to be the best. The parameter fitting was run for each capsule with 460 points in time using the thermal cycling profile shown in figure 6.12, using the temperature jump of run 4 from room to body temperature and the following 33 days of steady temperature.

For fitting the total observed time window, two variations of the Burger's model were used: 1/1/1 (as seen in fig. 3.9) and 1/2/1 where the first number is the number of pure springs elements, the second the number of combined spring-dampener elements and the third the pure dampener element. All elements are used in series.

The found parameter set was then applied to the fifth jump (fig. 6.12, last side) after a linear recalibration. For the linear recalibration the k_1 factor was adjusted to match the pressure increase during the temperature change from the initial room temperature to 99 % of the final body temperature. Then k_2 and k_3 were adjusted to maintain the original k_i/k_1 ratio. I1C3 and I2C4 stopped returning a stable signal and were therefore excluded from this chapter.

8.1.2 Results & Discussion

Figure 8.4 shows an example of the measured and simulated pressure error for one sensor with one pure spring, one combined spring-dampener and one pure dampener element (1/1/1) after fitting. Overall the calculated temperature-induced pressure error is reasonably replicated and the residual error remains within a ±1 mmHg window. However, in the initial phase after the temperature jump, the curvature of the measured and calculated pressure differ from each other (see fig. 8.5). The calculated pressure decay is slower at first, but takes more time to stabilize and undershoots the measured pressure at around 0.25 days. Further the trajectory of the calculated and simulated pressure differs in the following segment, leading to a steadily increasing difference between the measured and calculated pressures. The total and individual extension of the three elements is displayed in the bottom box. In the initial phase, where the total length of the system is increased (total length in the model corresponds to temperature), only the pure spring element reacts and extends almost as much as the total extension applied to the system. This extension of the pure spring element is the gradually and partially transferred to the combined spring-dampener element until the two springs reach their force equilibrium. From there on only the continued extension of the dampener allows the two other elements to slowly re-contract.

Figure 8.6 shows an example of the measured and simulated pressure error for one sensor with one pure spring, two combined spring-dampener and one pure dampener element (1/2/1) after fitting. Comparing fig. 8.7 with fig. 8.5 shows the much improved tracking of the pressure curve shape in the initial phase just after the temperature jump. The initial rapid pressure decay is replicated by the weaker dampener in the first combined spring-dampener element (S/D 1) and the transition into the region of slower decay is replicated by the stronger dampener in the second combined spring-dampener element (S/D 2). This can also be seen in the extension plot (fig. 8.5 and fig. 8.7, bottom). Where the SD 1 element of the 1/2/1 model extends faster and the S/D 2 element of the model 1/2/1 extends slower than the SD 1 element of the model 1/1/1. The improved tracking in the beginning then also results in more closely aligned trajectories in the later segment of the curve and therefore in a smaller overall error and a significantly reduced trend of the residual error. The individual residual error for each capsule after fitting can be found in figure A.17

Figure 8.8 shows an example of the measured and simulated pressure error for one sensor with one pure spring, two combined spring-dampener and one pure dampener element (1/2/1) on a segment of the recorded pressure, where no fitting was performed. Here only the simple linear recalibration of the spring constants previously extracted was performed. The calculated pressure and its curvature still follows the measured pressure closely. However, a small offset is visible. In figure 8.9 it can be seen that this offset originates at the beginning of the measurement and is caused by the slower initial decay of the calculated pressure, resulting in over correction of the measured pressure. The individual residual error for each capsule after fitting can be found in figure A.18.

The difference between the section where the model was fitted and the section where only the linear recalibration was performed becomes even more obvious in figure 8.10. After fitting in section 4, the residual error becomes comparable to the sensor's own uncertainty. In section 5 of figure 8.10, the previously observed overcorrection can be seen at the end of day one (fig. 8.10, section 5, 1i). In the following 10 day intervals, the added absolute residual error becomes less and is even corrected in interval 21i and 31i. In the last interval 41i, the change of error stabilizes. The stabilization in interval 41i indicates that the trajectories of the measured and calculated pressure are aligned. Thus a radical change of the residual error is not to be expected past 41t, considering that the measured and calculated pressure curves both flatten (i.e. the pressure change over time moves towards zero). The overall residual error (excluding outliers) after correction shown in figure 8.10, section 5, 41t is still well within ± 2 mmHg and for 11/20 capsules even within ± 1 mmHg (outliers shown in fig. A.16, fitted and corrected pressure profiles shown in fig. A.17 and fig. A.18).

Comparing figure A.16 to the uncorrected pressure errors in figure 6.15 shows a significant reduction of the temperature induced drift error.

Comparing this correction approach (fig. 8.10) to the approach described in the previous chapter (fig. 7.4) shows a similar spread amongst the final (41t) residual errors. The Burgers model based approach however is slightly biased towards under correction. The requirements of both approaches are shown in table 8.2

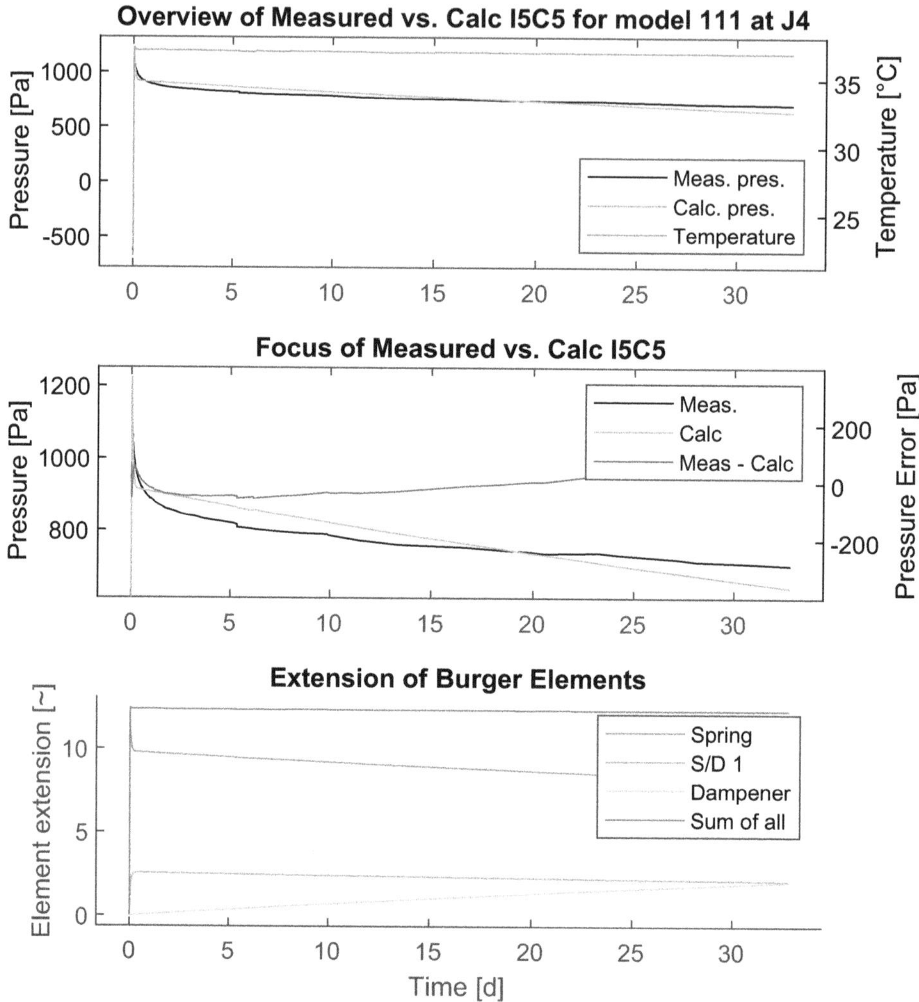

Figure 8.4: Top view: Overview of the measured and calculated pressures (left y-axis) and the applied temperature profile (right y-axis). Mid view: zoomed in view of the measured and calculated pressures (left y-axis) and the remaining temperature induced pressure error after correction (right y-axis). Bottom view: simulated extensions (x_i) of the total and individual components of the Burgers model.

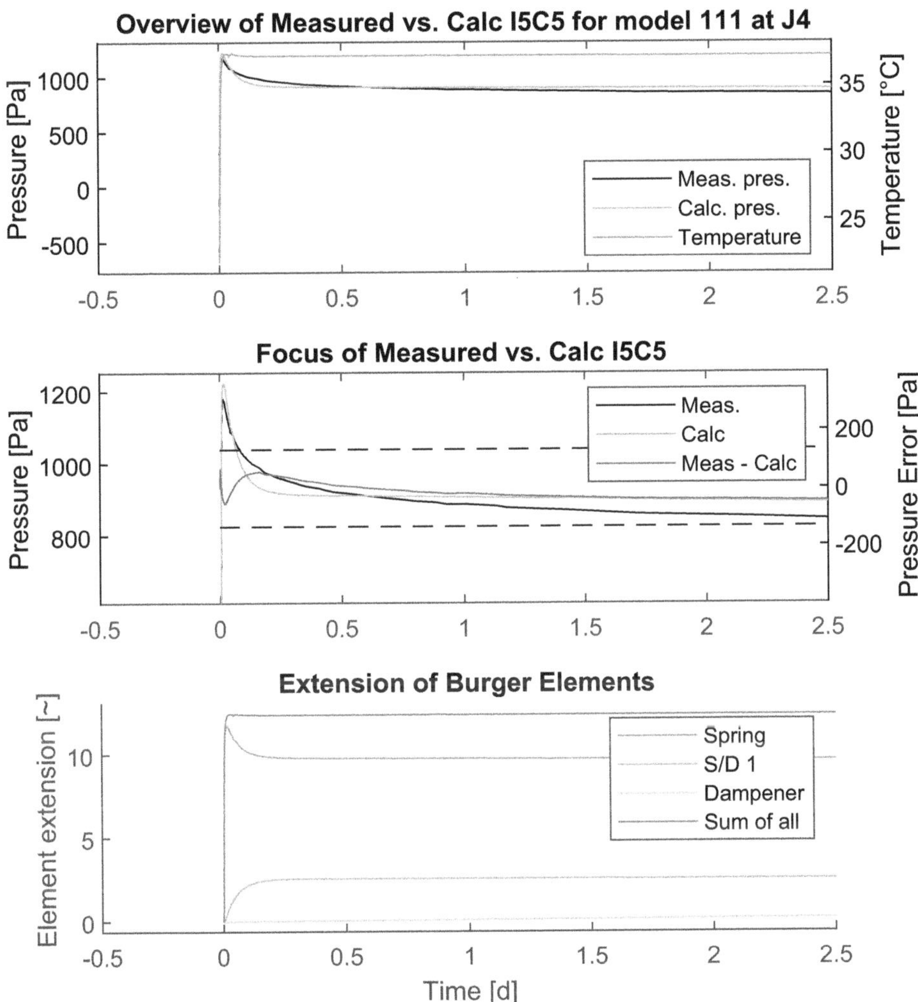

Figure 8.5: Zoomed in view of fig. 8.4. Top view: Overview of the measured and calculated pressures (left y-axis) and the applied temperature profile (right y-axis). Mid view: zoomed in view of the measured and calculated pressures (left y-axis) and the remaining temperature induced pressure error after correction (right y-axis). Bottom view: simulated extensions of the total and individual components of the Burgers model.

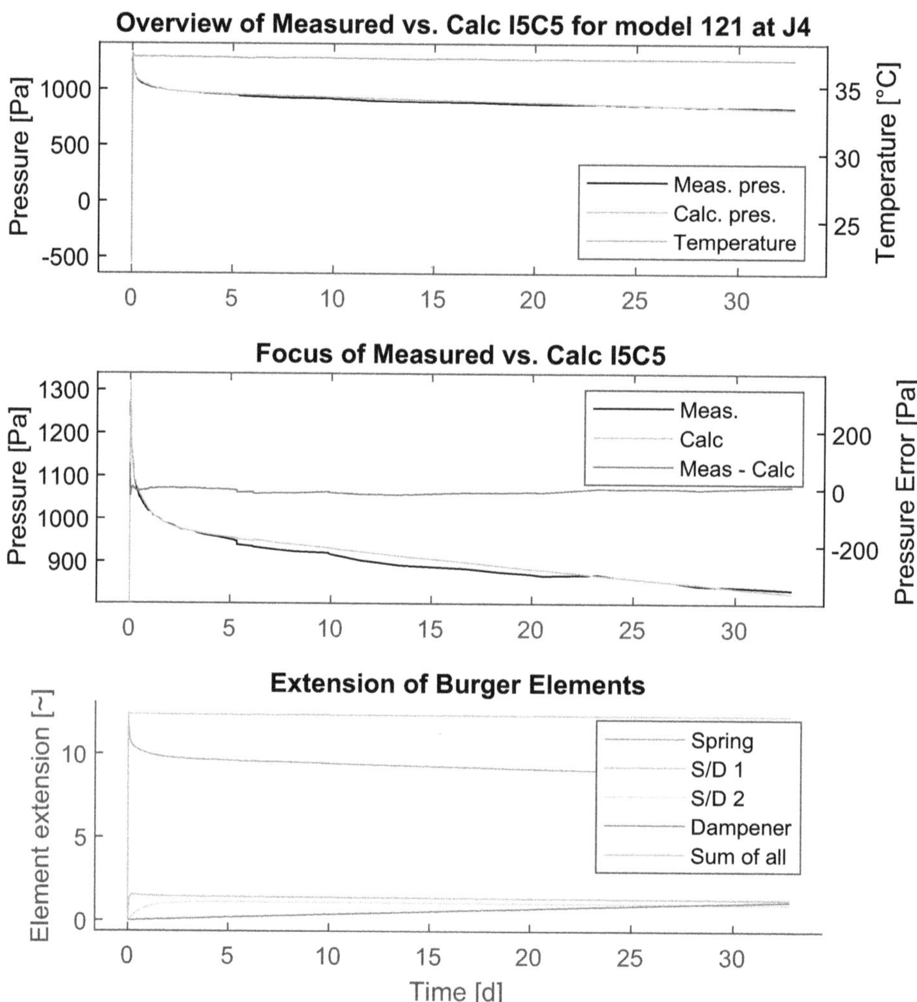

Figure 8.6: Top view: Overview of the measured and calculated pressures (left y-axis) and the applied temperature profile (right y-axis). Mid view: zoomed in view of the measured and calculated pressures (left y-axis) and the remaining temperature induced pressure error after correction (right y-axis). Bottom view: simulated extensions of the total and individual components of the Burgers model.

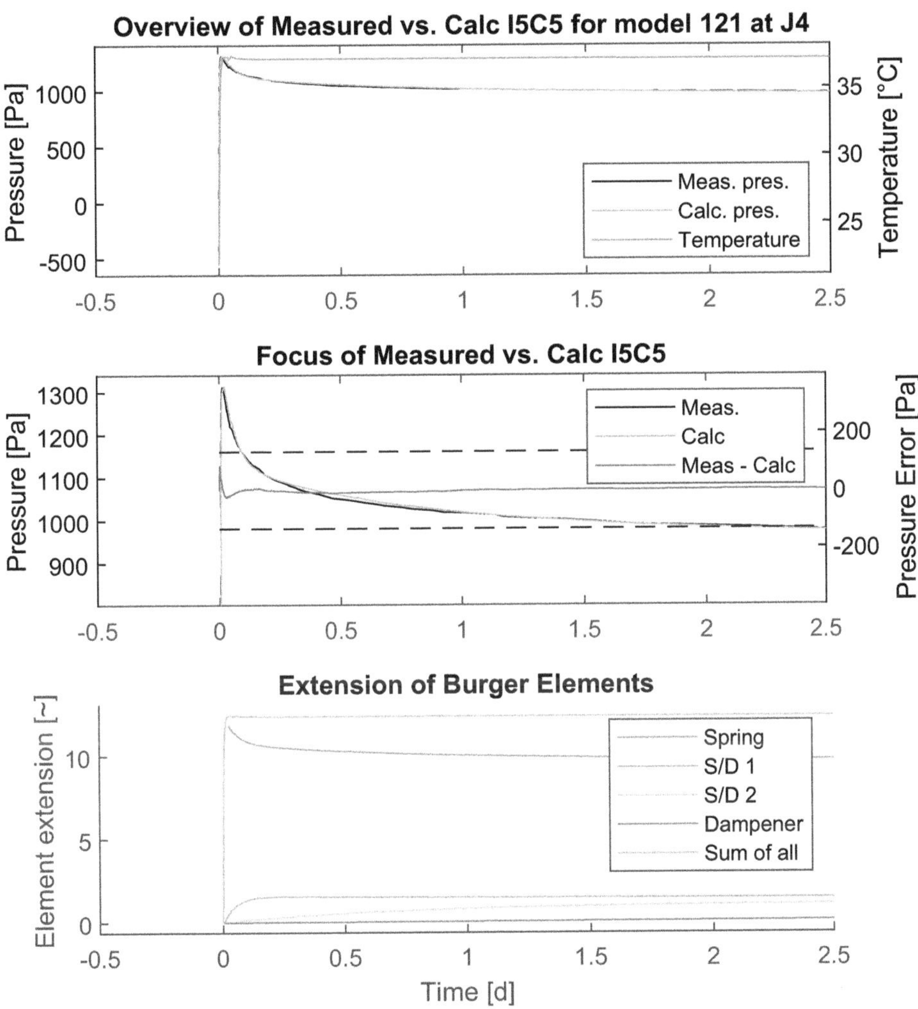

Figure 8.7: Zoomed in view of fig. 8.6. Top view: Overview of the measured and calculated pressures (left y-axis) and the applied temperature profile (right y-axis). Mid view: zoomed in view of the measured and calculated pressures (left y-axis) and the remaining temperature induced pressure error after correction (right y-axis). Bottom view: simulated extensions of the total and individual components of the Burgers model.

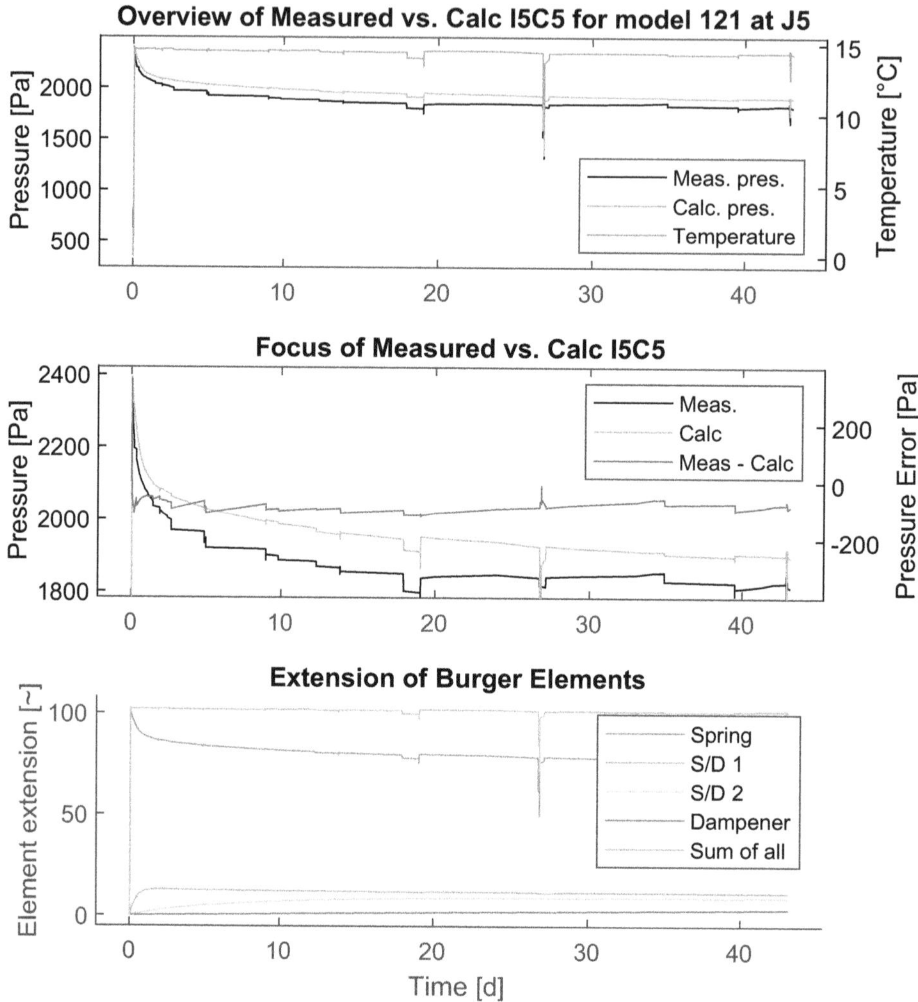

Figure 8.8: Top view: Overview of the measured and calculated pressures (left y-axis) and the applied temperature profile (right y-axis). Mid view: zoomed in view of the measured and calculated pressures (left y-axis) and the remaining temperature induced pressure error after correction (right y-axis). Bottom view: simulated extensions of the total and individual components of the Burgers model.

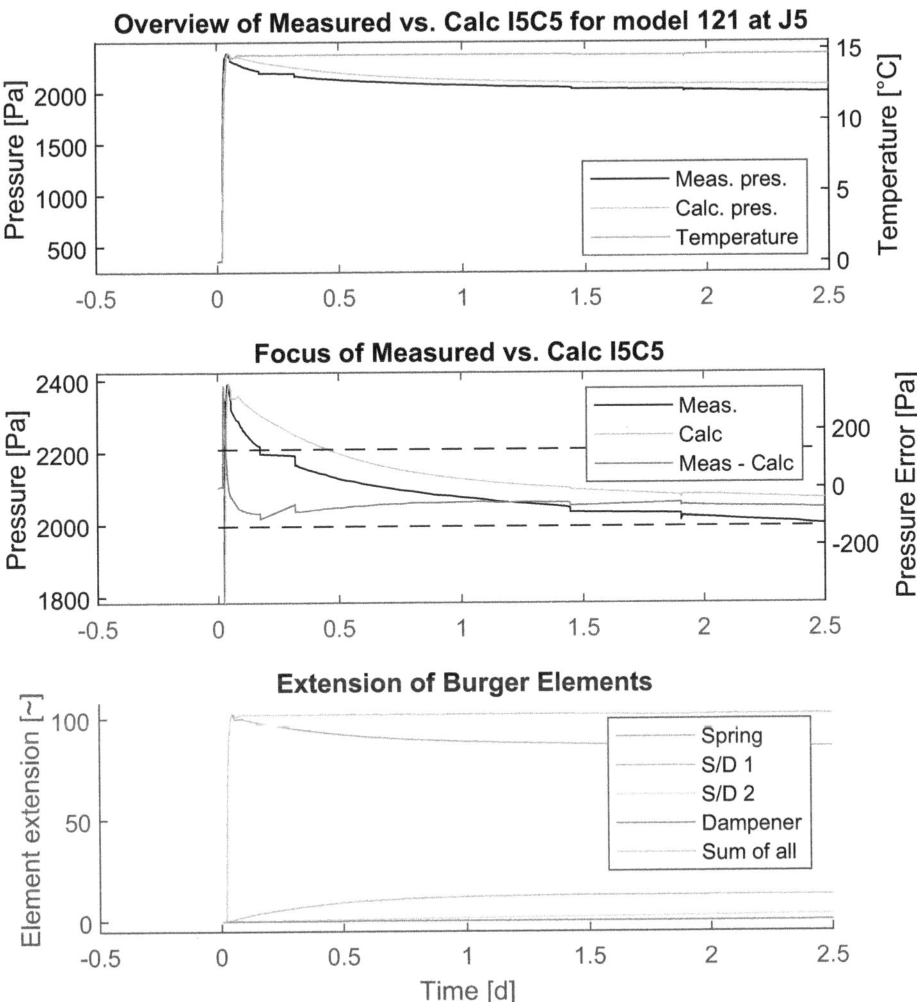

Figure 8.9: Zoomed in view of fig. 8.8. Top view: Overview of the measured and calculated pressures (left y-axis) and the applied temperature profile (right y-axis). Mid view: zoomed in view of the measured and calculated pressures (left y-axis) and the remaining temperature induced pressure error after correction (right y-axis). Bottom view: simulated extensions of the total and individual components of the Burgers model.

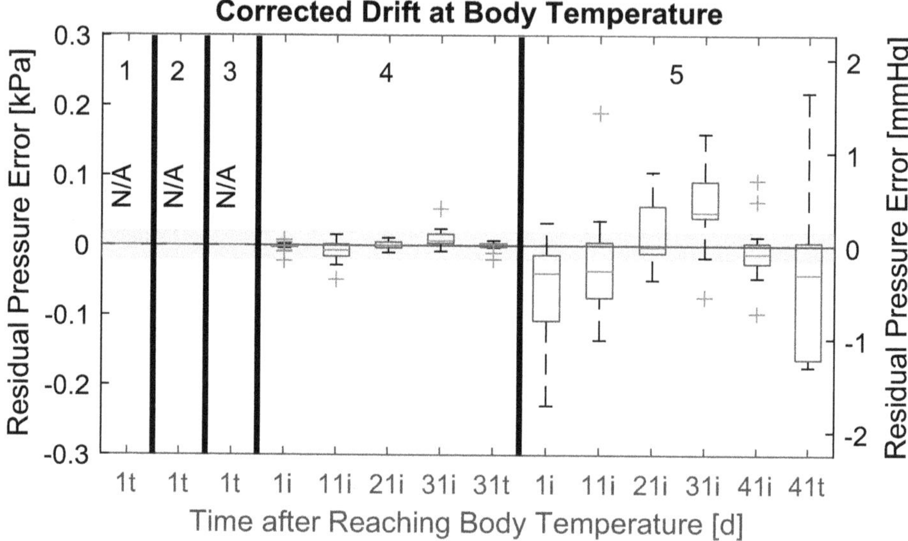

Figure 8.10: Residual error after drift correction with the Burgers model based algorithm (1/2/1). For the first day, then for intervals of 10 d and the total duration. The temperature jump of run 4 was used for fitting and extracting the model parameters for each sensor individually. the section "5" shows the residual error after correction based on the previously acquired parameter set and a linear recalibration. The orange (central band) area shows the sensor's uncertainty range. All outliers visible in fig. A.16.

Table 8.2: List of requirements for both correction approaches.

Requirement	Two-Sensor	Burgers Model
Nr. of sensors	2+	1
Pre-implantation	pressure transmission	Algorithm teach-in
At implantation	2 point calibration	2 point calibration

8.1.3 Conclusion

The model 1/2/1 was shown to replicate the temperature induced pressure error excellently after fitting. The transfer of the fitted parameter sets to a following temperature jump requires a linear recalibration, but results in an error reduction of similar quality to the approach described in the previous chapter, without the requirement of an additional sensor. The stabilization of the residual error promises a low residual error drift during long term application. However, it might be more suitable to use this correction only for the initial time period after implantation since the temperature induced pressure error itself stabilizes over time.

9 In-Vivo Experiment

A colored version of this chapter is available at: https://doi.org/10.3929/ethz-b-000702759

9.1 Animal Trial with Catheter Tip Pressure Sensor Reference

Implant 4 was successfully implanted in three acute animal trials and did not show signs of lessened functionality. Here the results of the fourth trial (second trial with this implant, see table A.3) are shown, where the implantation was successful and the pressures measured by the implant could be compared to a measurement taken by a catheter tip pressure sensor placed in the blood stream near the capsules.

9.1.1 Materials & Methods

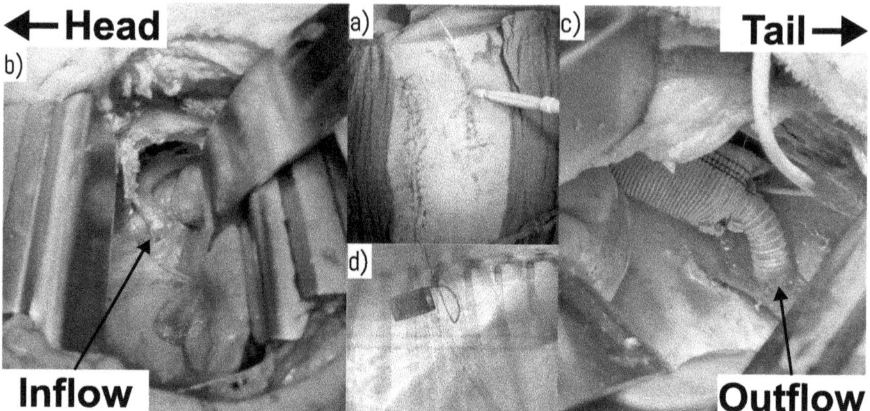

Figure 9.1: Photographic and x-ray images of the implant after implantation. a) Surgery site after complete implantation. b) View through the left incision, showing the proximal anastomosis, c) View through the right incision, showing the distal anastomosis, d) X-ray image of the implant in the ribcage.

Implant 4 was implanted in parallel to the aorta as can be seen in figure 9.1 via two incisions with 2 ribs in-between. A catheter tip absolute pressure sensor (SPR-524, Millar, USA), inserted via carotis communis, was placed in the inflow graft (proximal) of the implant. The pressure measurements of the 6 internal implant sensors were recorded by a python program during the surgery. Post explantation, the data recorded by the catheter tip was slightly stretched in time to correct a small time logging difference between the implant and catheter system by matching a pressure peak at the beginning and the end of the measurements. Furthermore, pressure data from the catheter tip was interpolated to match the implant's recording frequency. After that a line was fitted to the catheter pressure vs. sensor pressure plot and the line's parameter were used to calibrate the sensor's offset and sensitivity to that of the catheter sensor (see fig. A.19 and fig A.20) using:

$$p_{calib}(t) = a * p_{rec}(t) + b; \tag{9.1}$$

where $p_{calib}(t)$ is the calibrated sensor pressure, $p_{rec}(t)$ is the as-recorded sensor pressure, and a and b are the line's parameters. The maximal and minimal pressure values of each pulse were extracted using an automated Matlab script and compared.

9.1.2 Results & Discussion

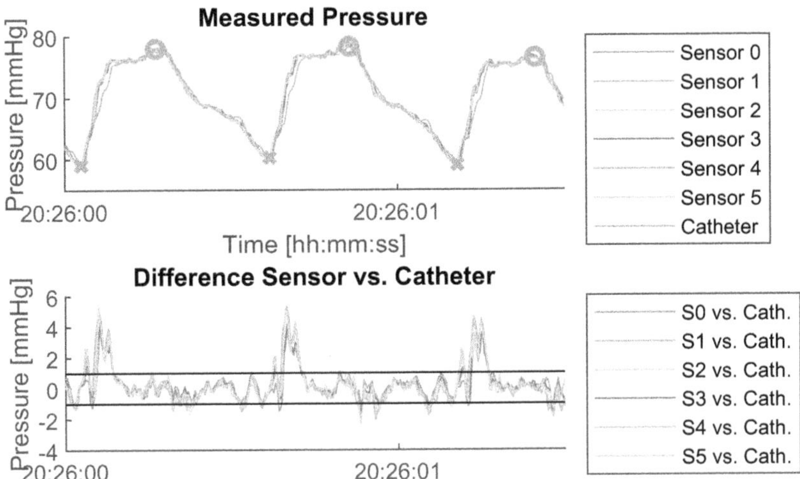

Figure 9.2: Section of the recorded data by the six capsules of the implant and the catheter tip sensor during the 4th animal trial and the difference between each capsule and the catheter tip sensor. The o mark the detected systole and the x mark the detected diastole.

Figure 9.2 (top) shows pressure recorded by the six internal sensors after calibration and the pressure recorded by the catheter tip sensor. The bottom plot shows the difference between each sensor and the reference. The excellent agreement of all six sensors amongst each other is immediately visible as well as the good agreement with the reference. Only at rising edge of the signal shows a deviation between the implants sensors and the catheter. In this region of fast pressure change, the sensors show a slightly earlier rise than the catheter. This could partially have been caused by a small time shift between the implant and the catheter. However, the rising slope of the catheter also differs in shape from the ones measured by the implant sensors. The positioning of the catheter sensor in the elastic graft, before the entrance to the rigid implant might also have influenced this highly dynamic region. In the region of interest for VAD control, the maximal and minimal pressures of each pulse however, the agreement between the catheter and implant is affected less. Figure 9.3 shows the distribution of the deviation between each implant capsule and the catheter sensor at the maximum and minimum of each pulse. With exception of a few outliers, the pressures recorded by the implant match the pressures recorded by the catheter sensor within a ± 1 mmHg window. Figure 9.4 shows the deviation of the measured pressure of the implant sensors to their mean recorded pressure for each maximum and minimum per pulse. The distribution is significantly smaller, showing the excellent internal agreement of the sensors.

The calibration factors (fig. A.20) used here show significant deviations. It is assumed that this was caused by erroneous readout software. The unedited recorded data (fig. A.21) shows sudden scaling and offset changes in-between measurement blocks, which remain for the duration of the block and sometimes extend to the next. This behaviour was not observed in later animal trials where an updated python readout software was used. Nevertheless, the shape of the pressure wave was retained in the quality discussed above. Outside of this calibration, which in essence is the pressure transmission correction (sec. 7.1), but replacing the in-vivo reference sensor with the catheter tip sensor. Drift and TCS had a neglectable impact, due to the short time window and stable temperature during the recording therefore no other of the correction methods detailed above had to be employed.

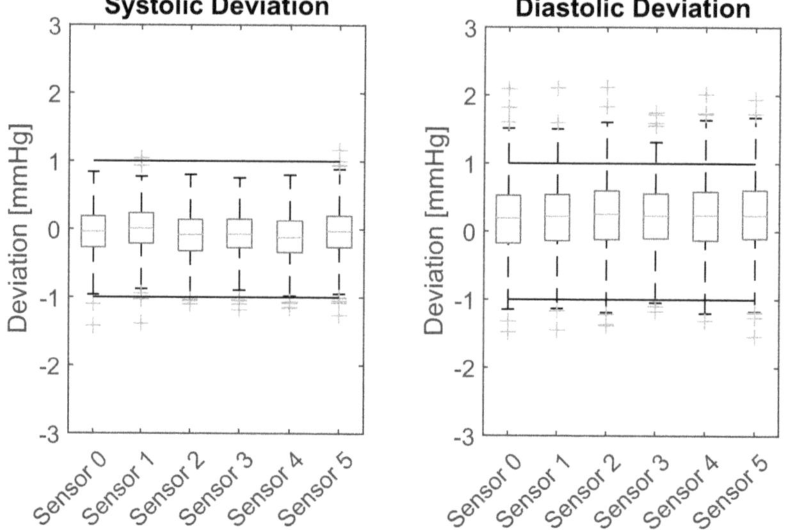

Figure 9.3: Deviation between the capsules and the catheter tip sensor at systole and diastole.

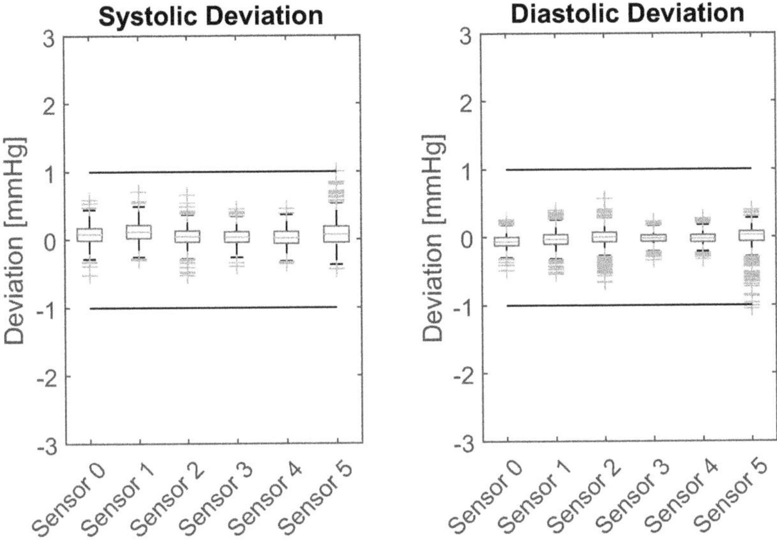

Figure 9.4: Deviation between the capsules and the mean of all capsules at systole and diastole. The agreement amongst each other is better then compared to the catheter tip sensor. (see fig. 9.3)

9.1.3 Conclusion

The failure free operation of the same implant in 4 animal trials confirms the applicability and reliability of the design for animal trials. The acquired data and its internal agreement in the discussed animal trial display the reproducible pressure acquisition of the implant. With the readout software issue solved, this places the implant and readout setup in a good position for future animal trials.

10 Conclusion and Outlook

In this thesis an MSPSE for continuous blood pressure measurement was designed, produced and integrated in a testing platform for long-term animal trials. The developed production process addresses systematic error sources, especially with respect to drift. The produced devices demonstrate the feasibility of the process as well as the translatability towards VADs. The characterization of the devices revealed further path ways towards trueness improvement by systematic error correction, also with respect to drift.

10.1 Summary & Accomplishments

The state of the art review demonstrates the multitude of potential benefits of autonomous VAD operation and that the lack of suitable sensor systems prevents this revolutionary development of VAD technology. Previously explored approaches are discussed and the particularly promising approach of integrating an MSD in the coating of an inflow cannula was chosen as a starting point for this thesis.

The concept of an MSPSE with its functional components is explained and the influence of its design parameters on the trueness of the resulting device are laid out, including additional considerations for the viscoelastic nature of the chosen MSD material. The key concept for high trueness is found to be a minimized pressure difference across the MSD, both during fabrication and later during operation. The most significant challenge to this concept in the fabrication process was found to be assembly induced internal overpressure, created by the final sealing step. For the operation it was found to be the temperature induced pressure increase during the implantation of the device.

Minimization of assembly induced internal overpressure was achieved by a minimal injection volume sealing process, which allows excess enclosed pressure transmission fluid to exit during the sealing. Temperature cross sensitivity was addressed by maximizing the membrane size to pressure transmission fluid ratio. For this purpose, two methods, enabling arbitrary MSD shapes unconstrained by the pressure transmission channel, were developed and the superior solution was employed to manufacture the testing platforms and inflow cannulas.

The produced MSPSEs showed excellent pressure transmission and TCSs within the target range for uncorrected operation around body temperature. However, the TCS from room to body temperature was found to be larger than desired, likely due to the curvature of the MSDs which was inherited from the inner diameter of the implantable testing platforms.

The TCS and drift behaviour after a temperature increase to body temperature was studied and revealed a strong correlation between the initial temperature induced pressure increase and the systematic pressure decay thereafter. This correlation was exploited to drastically improve the trueness of the MSPSEs for sensor systems where at least two MSPSEs are available.

The Burgers model for viscoelastic materials was adapted to describe the measured temperature-pressure-time relation and found to be able to almost perfectly replicate it. Based on the developed model a second approach for correction of the TCS and drift behaviour after a temperature increase to body temperature was developed. This approach offers a solution for single-capsule systems at the cost of a slightly lower trueness, but still excellent overall accuracy.

One of the produced implantable testing platforms was successfully implanted in three animal trials and showed an excellent agreement of all included MSPSEs with a catheter tip mounted absolute pressure sensor, placed in the blood stream near the implant. The agreement of the sensor amongst each other was found to be even better, demonstrating the quality of the pressure transmission characteristic of the device.

In Summary, drift was identified as the main challenge amongst the existing systems in the literature and addressed at the design stage and in post processing. The existing MSD-in-coating approach was expanded by a method to control the shape of the MSD independently, enabling the reduction of TCS and therefore viscoelastic drift at the design stage. To further reduce drift, two potent solutions were developed showing that the drift in this system is predictable. These results show that accurate pressure sensing is achievable even while employing biocompatible polymers.

10.2 Discussion & Outlook

While the presented MSPSEs showed excellent pressure transmission in-vitro and in-vivo and the designed TCS for correction free operation around body temperature, the TCS from body to room temperature and the resulting pressure drift thereafter are larger than desired and require compensation in the current state of the device. A reduction of the curvature by either reducing the width of the MSD or increasing the inner diameter of the implant is expected to reduce the TCS from room temperature. The former approach would entail a reduction of the pressure transmission liquid volume, which seems feasible, especially considering advanced additive manufacturing technologies. This reduction would also naturally occur with the miniaturization of the MSPSE for future applications. The later approach, a larger inner diameter, while dictated by flow considerations of blood in the inflow cannula, is already the case in some VADs.

Furthermore, long term animal trials should be conducted to study the influence of extended blood contact on the exposed MSD.

11 List of Student Projects

B. Mueller, "Selective tio2 nanostructure removal for parylene-c membrane fabrication," Bachelor Thesis, 2019.

P. Martin, "Curved membrane design and fabrication," Master Thesis, 2019.

P. Mueller, "Miniaturization of an injection-volume optimized backside sealing," Bachelor Thesis, 2019.

R. Graf, "Optimization and miniaturization of a hermetic solder seal," Master Thesis, 2019.

I. Hutter, "Leakage assessment of a parylene-c/tio2-nanostructure interface," Bachelor Thesis, 2020.

I. Hutter, "Leakage assessment of a parylene-c/tio2-nanostructure interface," Bachelor Thesis, 2020.

S. Ruth, "Membrane Shape Dependant Temperature Cross-sensitivity," Research Internship, 2020.

12 List of Publications

12.0.1 Article

P.S. Ravaynia, F.C. Lombardo, S. Biendl, M.A. Dupuch, J. Keiser, A. Hierlemann, M.M. Modena, "Parallelized Impedance-Based Platform for Continuous Dose-Response Characterization of Antischistosomal Drugs," Adv Biosyst 4(7) (2020), doi: 10.1002/adbi.201900304.

K. Von Petersdorff-Campen, M.A. Dupuch, K. Magkoutas, C. Hierold, M. Schmid Daners, "Pressure and Bernoulli-based Flow Measurement via a Tapered Inflow VAD Cannula," IEEE Trans Biomed Eng PP (2021), doi: 10.1109/TBME.2021.3123983.

12.0.2 Oral Abstract

M. Dupuch, J. Kaemmel, A. Alogna, K. Reiter, N. Cesarovic, V. Stoessel, P. Ostach, V. Falk, C. Starck, C. Hierold, "Inflow Cannula Pressure Sensor for Autonomous Dynamic Ventricular Assist Device Control," Thorac Cardiovasc Surg 70(S 01) (2022) DGTHG-V46, doi: 10.1055/s-0042-1742840.

K. von Petersdorff-Campen, M.A. Dupuch, K. Magkoutas, C. Hierold, M.S. Daners, "BIO8: Cannula Add-On For Pressure And Flow Measurement In VADs," Asaio J 68(Supplement 2) (2022) 13, doi: 10.1097/01.mat.0000840768.20168.7a.

Curriculum Vitae

Personal Details

Name	DUPUCH, Matthias Alexander
Birth	12 05 1986, Chene-Bougeries, SWITZERLAND
Citizenship	Switzerland & France
Marital Status	Married

Education

02/2019 – 03/2023	**Micro and Nanosystems Group, ETH Zurich, Switzerland** PhD Dissertaion "'Implantable Pressure Sensor Encapsulation for Ventricular Assist Device Control"'
09/2014 – 04/2016	**Micro and Nanosystems Program, ETH Zurich, Switzerland** MSc Thesis "Characterization of the Batch Assembly Process of Singlewalled Carbon Nanotubes Utilizing Functionalized Single Strand DNA"
09/2008 – 02/2014	**Mechanical and Process Engineering Program, ETH Zurich, Switzerland** BSc Thesis "Characterization of Flame-Made SiO2 Nanoparticles for Toxicological Studies"

Work Experience

05/2016 – 02/2019	**Micro and Nanosystems Group, ETH Zurich, Switzerland** Scientific Assistant
03/2014 – 09/2014	**Tata Motors, Pune, India** Internship

Languages

German	Fluent
English	Fluent
French	Advanced

A Appendix A

A colored version of this chapter is available at: https://doi.org/10.3929/ethz-b-000702759

A.1 Implant Characterization

Appendix for ch. 6.

Table A.1: List of requirements for both correction approaches.

Implant Nr.	Characterized	Cause
1	yes	-
2	yes	-
3	no	PCB damaged before the step "Oil Fill", assembly aborted
4	yes	-
5	yes	-
6	no	faulty readout electronics, implant still functioning

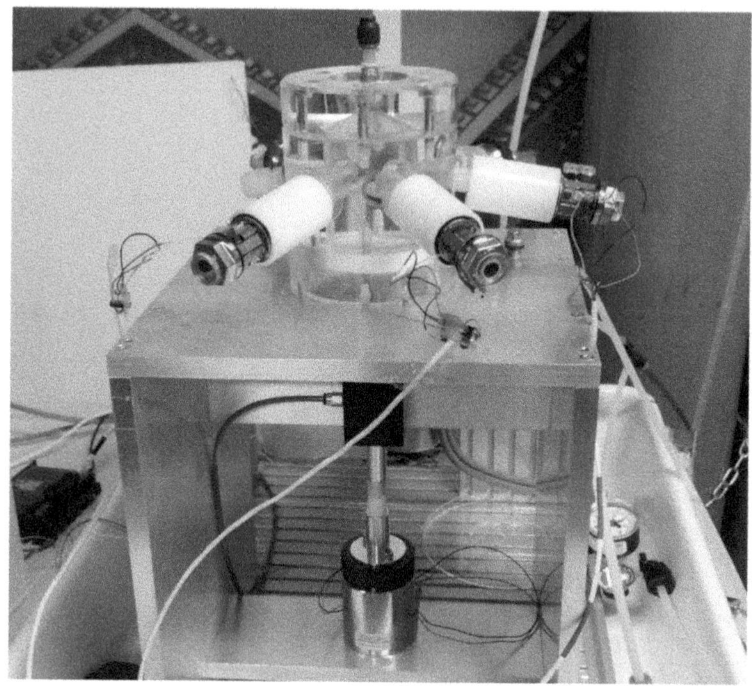

Figure A.1: Photography image of the pressure transmission testing station with three implants attached to it. The coil drive at the bottom is used to apply pressure inside the tank via transmission rod and flexible MSD. Setup from [40]

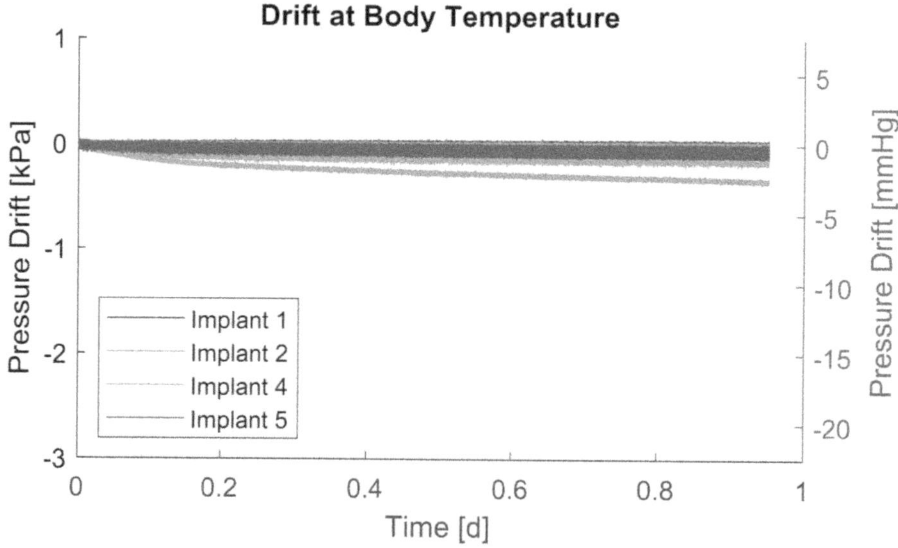

Figure A.2: Pressure drift after temperature jump over the course of 1 day. Run 1

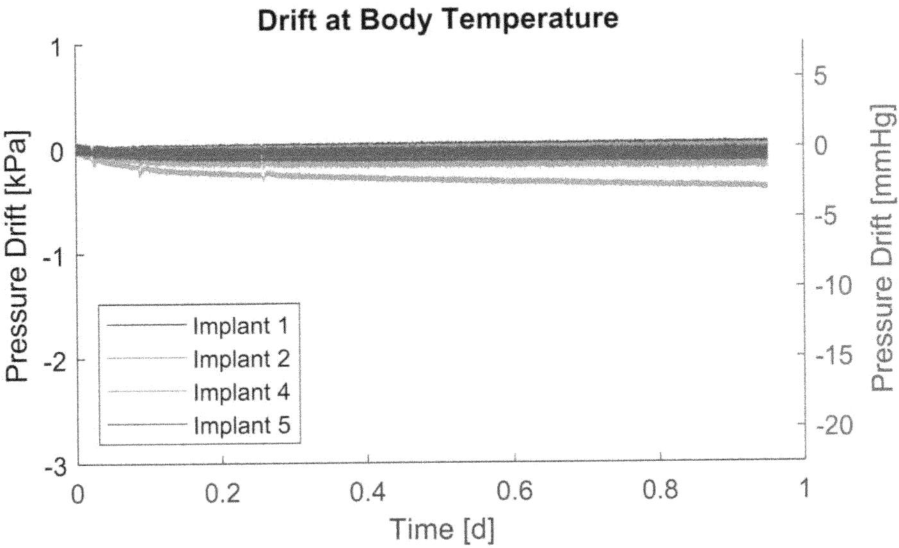

Figure A.3: Pressure drift after temperature jump over the course of 1 day. Run 2

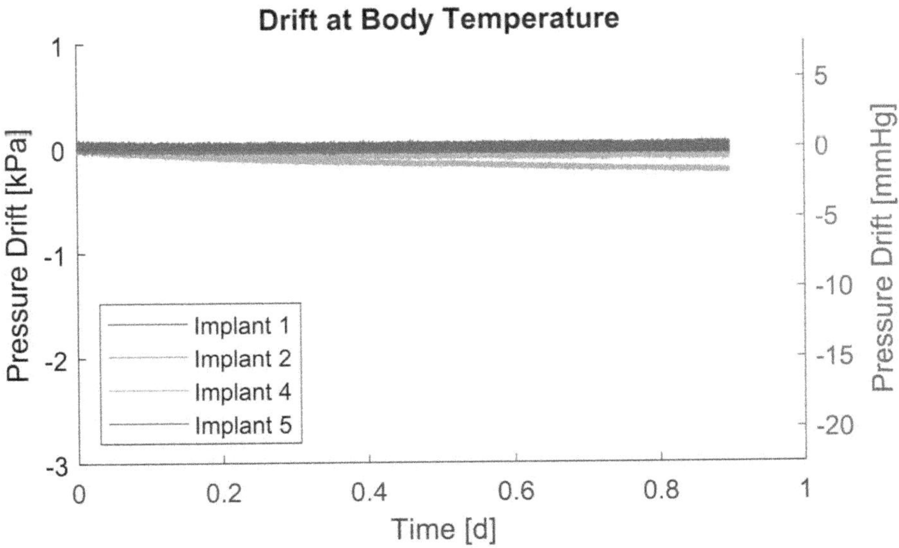

Figure A.4: Pressure drift after temperature jump over the course of 1 day. Run 3

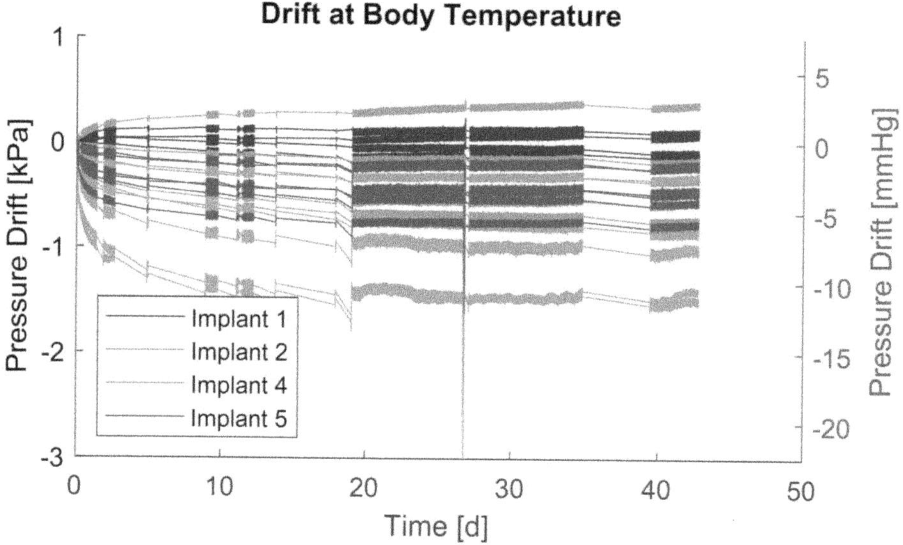

Figure A.5: Pressure drift after temperature jump over the course of 42.7 days. Run 5

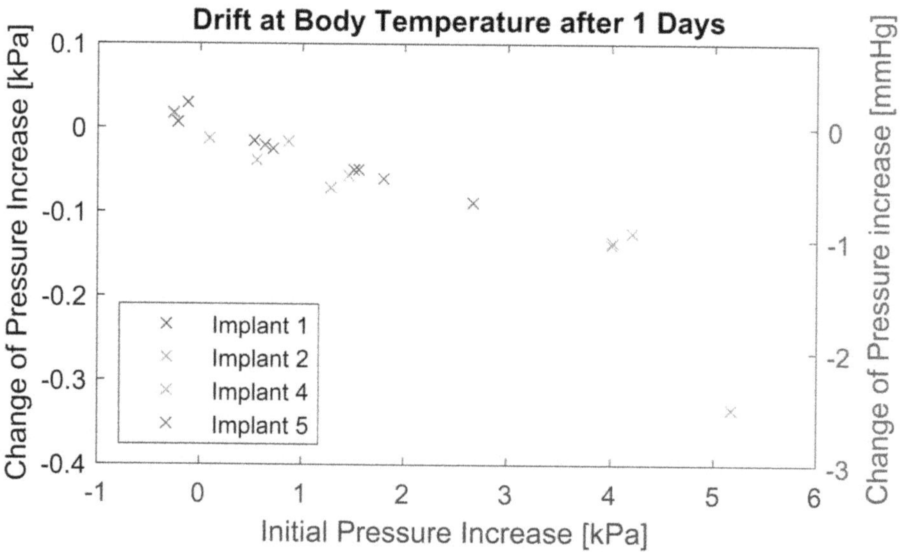

Figure A.6: Change or thermally induced pressure increase after 1 day in relation to the initial increase. Run 1

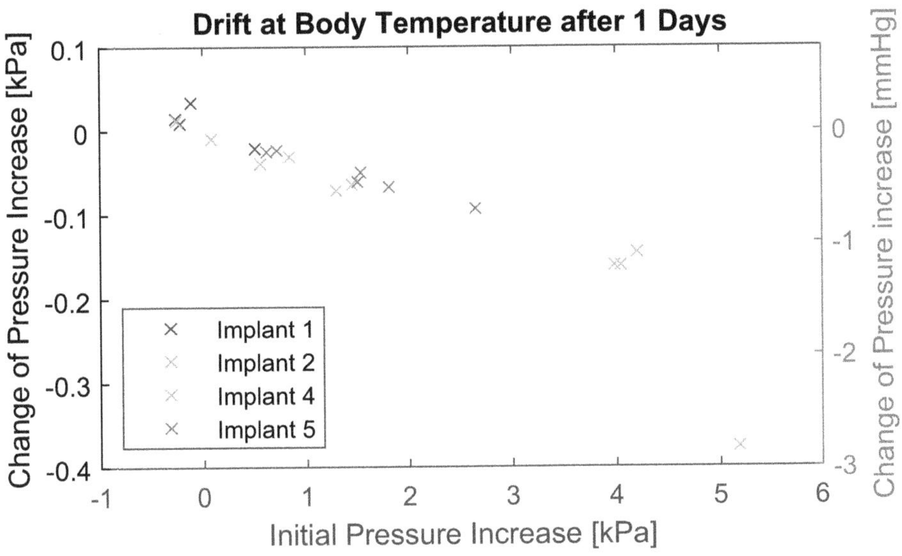

Figure A.7: Change or thermally induced pressure increase after 1 day in relation to the initial increase. Run 2

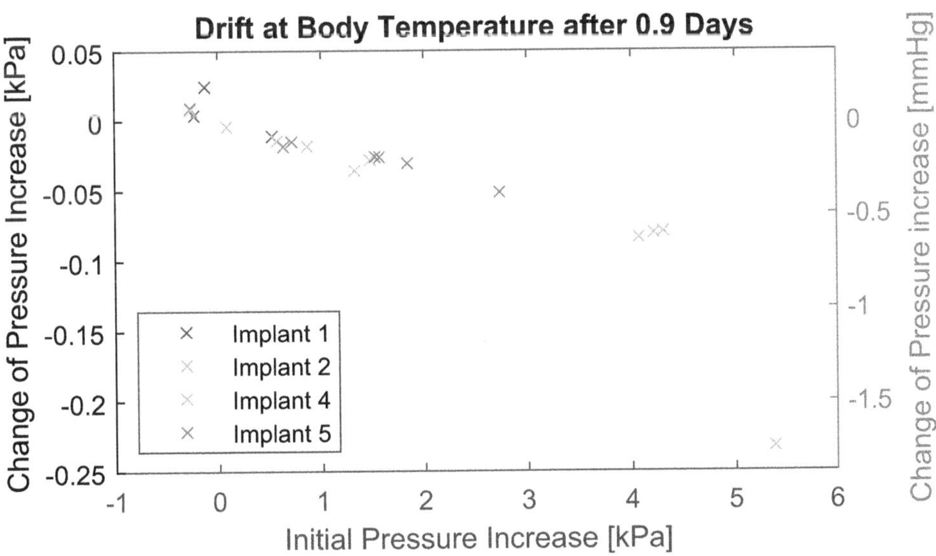

Figure A.8: Change or thermally induced pressure increase after 0.9 days in relation to the initial increase. Run 3

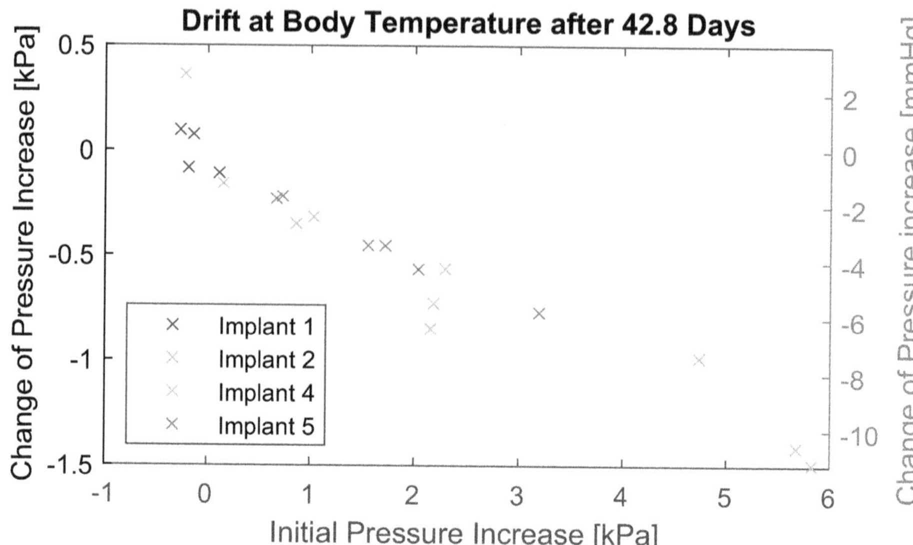

Figure A.9: Change or thermally induced pressure increase after 42.7 days in relation to the initial increase. Run 5

A.2 Error Correction

Appendix for ch. 7.
Starting with:

$$p_{1,d-corr}(t) = p_1(t) - \Delta p_{ref,th}(t)\frac{\Delta p_{1,th}}{\Delta p_{ref,th}} \tag{A.1}$$

and solving:

$$p_{2,d-corr}(t) = p_2(t) - \Delta p_{ref,th}(t)\frac{\Delta p_{2,th}}{\Delta p_{ref,th}} \tag{A.2}$$

for $p_{ref,th}$:

$$\Delta p_{ref,th}(t) = (p_2(t) - p_{2,d-corr}(t))\frac{\Delta p_{ref,th}}{\Delta p_{2,th}} \tag{A.3}$$

placing eq. A.3 in eq. A.1:

$$p_{1,d-corr}(t) = p_1(t) - (p_2(t) - p_{2,d-corr}(t))\frac{\Delta p_{ref,th}}{\Delta p_{2,th}}\frac{\Delta p_{1,th}}{\Delta p_{ref,th}} \tag{A.4}$$

solving for $p_{1,d-corr}(t)$ (the ambient pressure (e.g. blood pressure), therefore equal to $p_{2,d-corr}(t)$):

$$p_{1,d-corr}(t)(1 - \frac{\Delta p_{1,th}}{\Delta p_{2,th}}) = p_1(t) - p_2(t)\frac{\Delta p_{1,th}}{\Delta p_{2,th}} \tag{A.5}$$

$$p_{1,d-corr}(t) = \frac{p_1(t) - p_2(t)\frac{\Delta p_{1,th}}{\Delta p_{2,th}}}{(1 - \frac{\Delta p_{1,th}}{\Delta p_{2,th}})} \tag{A.6}$$

$$p_{1,d-corr}(t) = \frac{p_1(t)\Delta p_{2,th} - p_2(t)\Delta p_{1,th}}{(\Delta p_{2,th} - \Delta p_{1,th})} \tag{A.7}$$

$$p_{1,d-corr}(t) = \frac{p_1(t) * \Delta p_{2,th} - p_2(t) * \Delta p_{1,th}}{\Delta p_{2,th} - \Delta p_{1,th}} \tag{A.8}$$

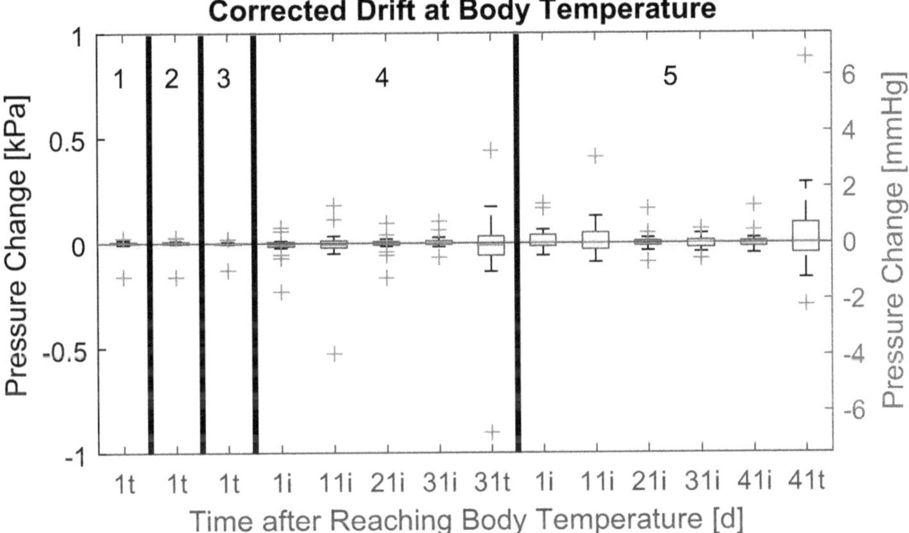

Figure A.10: Residual error after drift correction. For the first day, then for intervals of 10 d and the total duration. Zoomed out version.

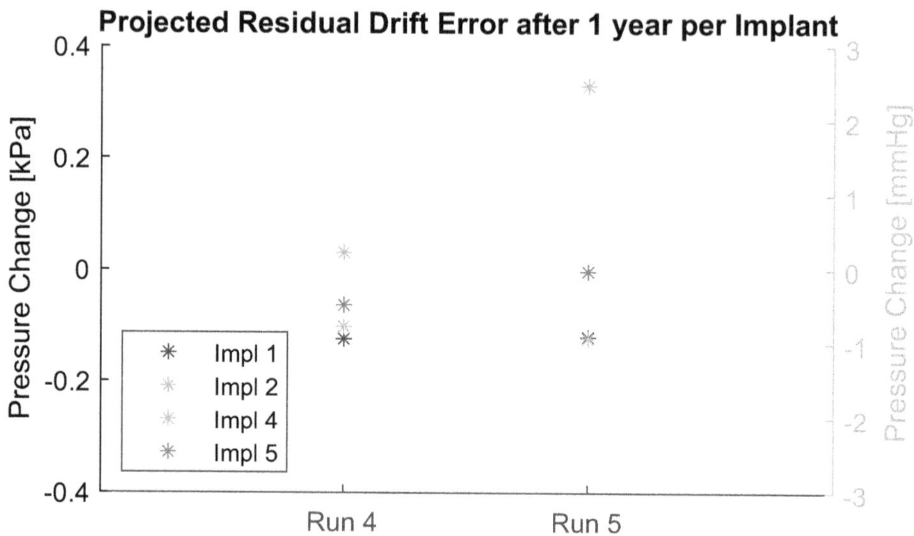

Figure A.11: Drift error projection based on the implant-wise averaged drift after omission of the least disagreeing MSPSE.

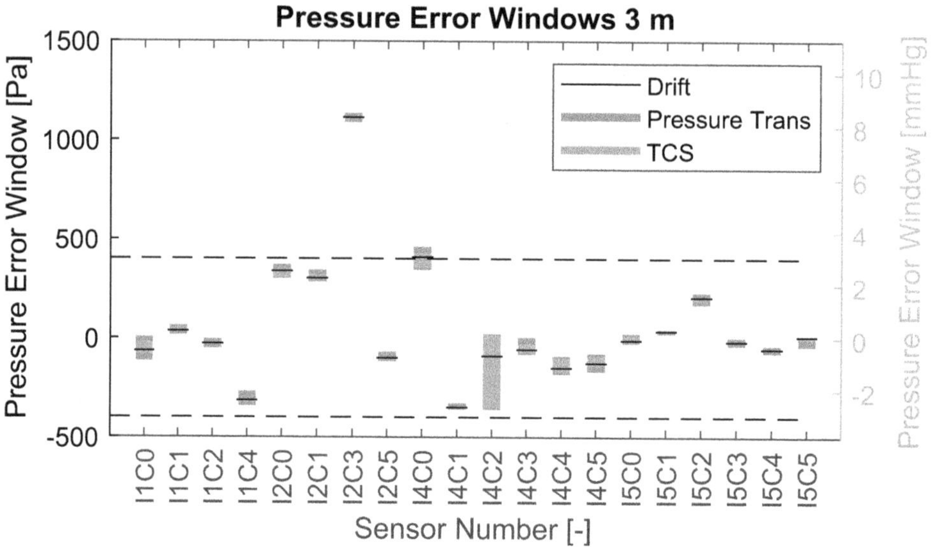

Figure A.12: Drift error window projection for each sensor after 3 months.

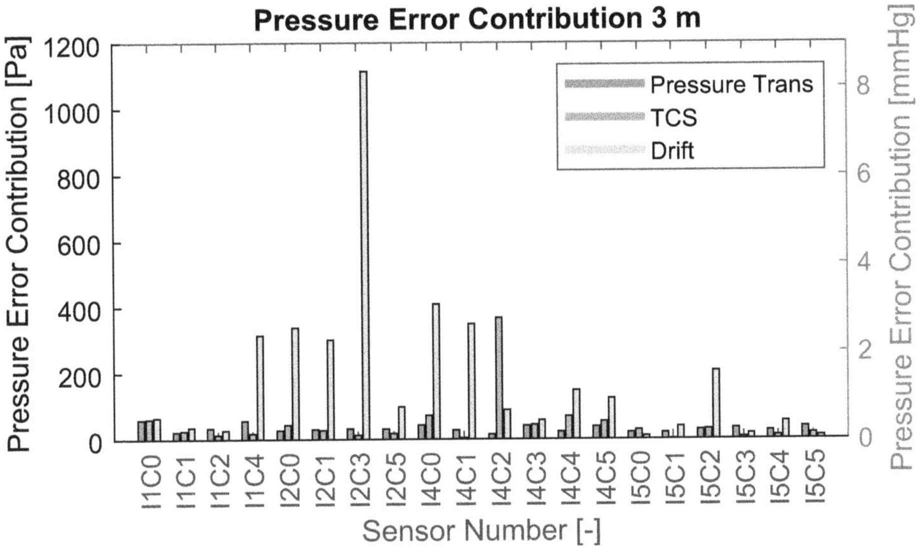

Figure A.13: Projected error source comparison for 3 months.

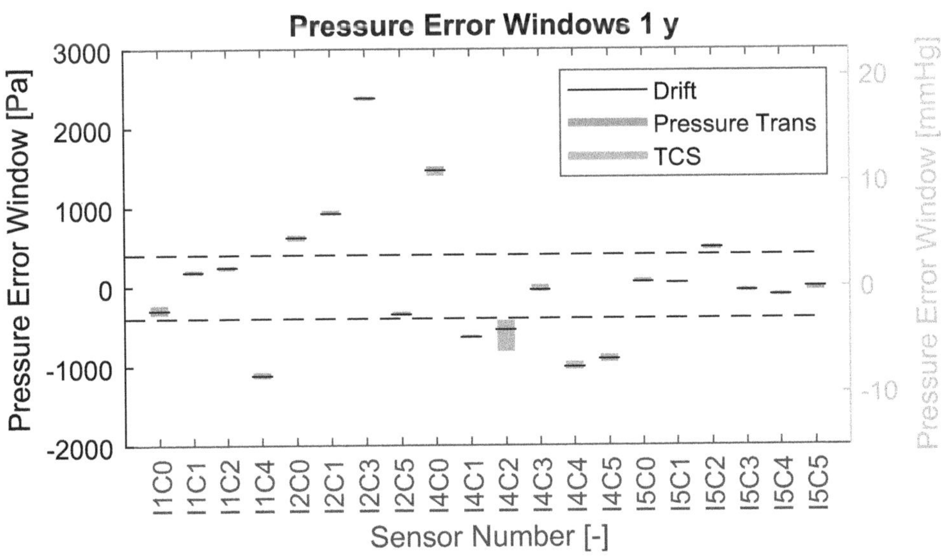

Figure A.14: Drift error window projection for each sensor after 1 year.

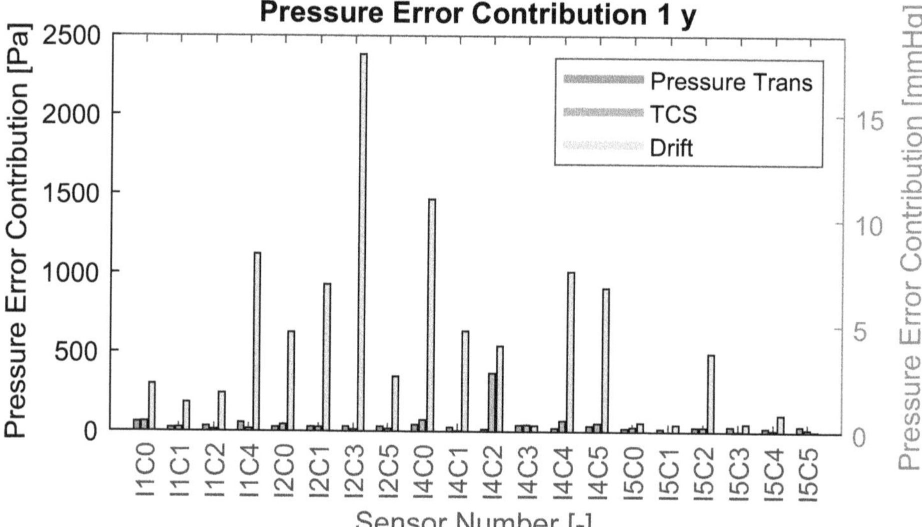

Figure A.15: Projected error source comparison for 1 year.

A.3 Model Based TCS Correction (Burgers Model)

Appendix for ch. 8. Starting with:

$$X(t_{j+1}) = \sum_{1}^{n} x_i(t_{j+1}) \tag{A.9}$$

and

$$F(t_{j+1}) = k_i x_i(t_{j+1}) + d_i \frac{x_i(t_{j+1}) - x_i(t_j)}{t_{j+1} - t_j} \tag{A.10}$$

Solving eq. A.10 for $x_i(t_{j+1})$:

$$F(t_{j+1}) = x_i(t_{j+1})\left(k_i + \frac{d_i}{t_{j+1} - t_j}\right) - \frac{d_i}{t_{j+1} - t_j} x_i(t_j) \tag{A.11}$$

$$x_i(t_{j+1})\left(k_i + \frac{d_i}{t_{j+1} - t_j}\right) = F(t_{j+1}) + \frac{d_i}{t_{j+1} - t_j} x_i(t_j) \tag{A.12}$$

$$x_i(t_{j+1}) = \frac{F(t_{j+1}) + \frac{d_i}{t_{j+1}-t_j} x_i(t_j)}{k_i + \frac{d_i}{t_{j+1}-t_j}} \tag{A.13}$$

Replacing $x_i(t_{j+1})$ in eq. A.9:

$$X(t_{j+1}) = \sum_{1}^{n} \frac{F(t_{j+1}) + \frac{d_i}{t_{j+1}-t_j} x_i(t_j)}{k_i + \frac{d_i}{t_{j+1}-t_j}} \tag{A.14}$$

and solving for $F(t_{j+1})$:

$$X(t_{j+1}) = \sum_{1}^{n} \frac{F(t_{j+1})}{k_i + \frac{d_i}{t_{j+1}-t_j}} + \sum_{1}^{n} \frac{\frac{d_i}{t_{j+1}-t_j} x_i(t_j)}{k_i + \frac{d_i}{t_{j+1}-t_j}} \tag{A.15}$$

$$\sum_{1}^{n} \frac{F(t_{j+1})}{k_i + \frac{d_i}{t_{j+1}-t_j}} = X(t_{j+1}) - \sum_{1}^{n} \frac{\frac{d_i}{t_{j+1}-t_j} x_i(t_j)}{k_i + \frac{d_i}{t_{j+1}-t_j}} \tag{A.16}$$

$$F(t_{j+1}) = \frac{X(t_{j+1}) - \sum_1^n \frac{\frac{d_i}{t_{j+1}-t_j} x_i(t_j)}{k_i + \frac{d_i}{t_{j+1}-t_j}}}{\sum_1^n \frac{1}{k_i + \frac{d_i}{t_{j+1}-t_j}}} \tag{A.17}$$

and finally replacing the model quantities X and F with T_{lin} and p_{calc}

$$p_{Calc}(t_{j+1}) = \frac{T_{lin}(t_{j+1}) - \sum_1^n \frac{\frac{d_i}{t_{j+1}-t_j} x_i(t_j)}{k_i + \frac{d_i}{t_{j+1}-t_j}}}{\sum_1^n \frac{1}{k_i + \frac{d_i}{t_{j+1}-t_j}}} \tag{A.18}$$

Now the model variables x_i can be found with eq. A.13

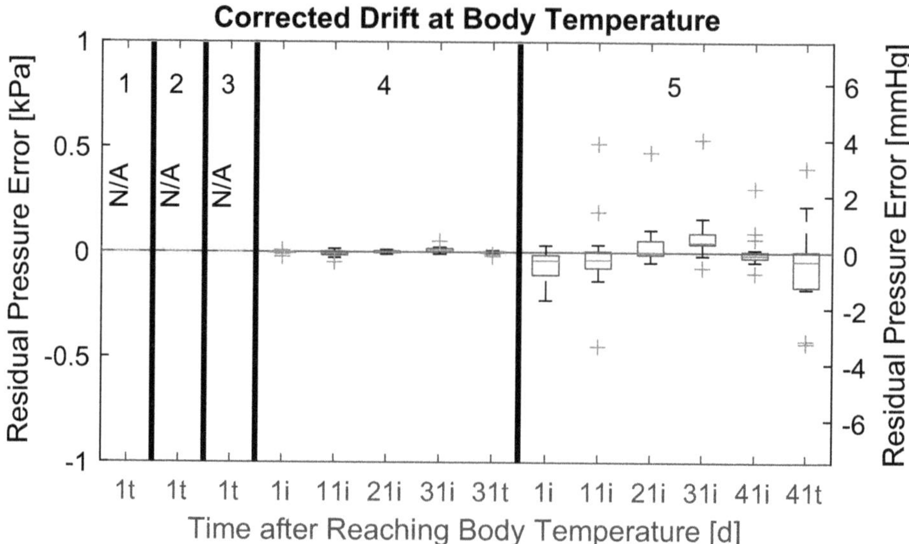

Figure A.16: Residual error after drift correction with the Burgers model based algorithm. For the first day, then for intervals of 10 d and the total duration. The temperature jump "4" was used for fitting and extracting the model parameters for each sensor individually. the section "5" shows the residual error after correction based on the previously acquired parameter set and a linear recalibration. The orange (central band) area shows the sensor's uncertainty range. 2 outliers in section 5, 21i at 4.6 kPa and 41t at 1.8 kPa are outside of the shown window.

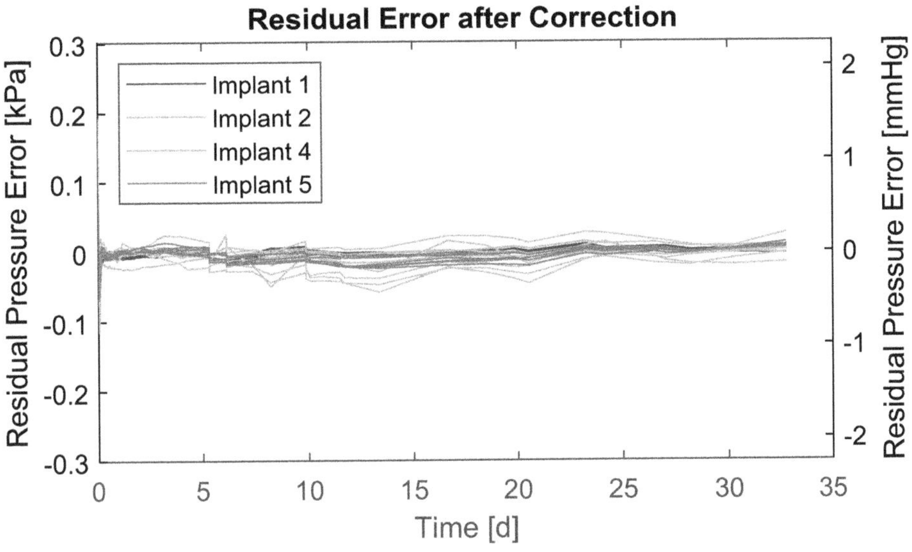

Figure A.17: Residual error after drift correction with the Burgers model based algorithm on section "4" where the parameters were fitted.

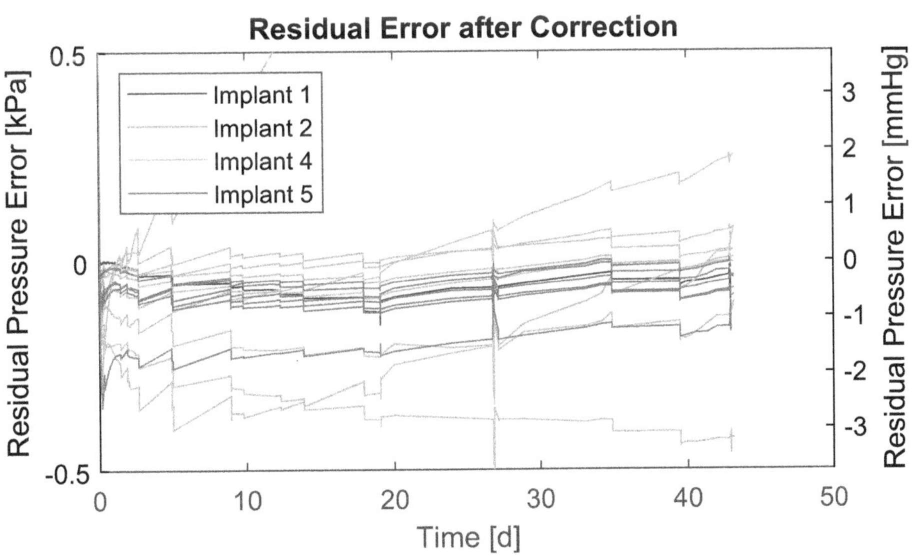

Figure A.18: Residual error after drift correction with the Burgers model based algorithm on section "5" where the parameters were not re-fitted and only a linear calibration was performed.

Table A.2: k and d values for each capsule for the 1/2/1 model as obtained from the fitting process. d = 0 indicates a pure spring element, k = 0 indicates a pure dampener element.

	Element 1	Element 2	Element 3	Element 4
I1C0	1.522	2.9308	31.9185	0
I1C0	0	4.8982	3191851.5462	23821417.6704
I1C1	1.2367	20.4326	144.9136	0
I1C1	0	547137.9724	7436357.4449	3774208.29
I1C2	1.2387	5.7527	3.7298	0
I1C2	0	48301.9645	876753.2631	3817693.1212
I1C3	1.1868	7.2273	11.1176	0
I1C3	0	59928.4355	1268248.4065	6730090.1545
I1C4	1.4215	3.14	172.4256	0
I1C4	0	0.56222	674917.1667	8187279.7441
I2C0	1.3332	5.4641	7.5961	0
I2C0	0	38257.1652	939217.2072	3910147.8642
I2C1	1.282	3.9585	12.2082	0
I2C1	0	1.7267	195724084362340.9	10206010.1448
I2C3	1.2939	5.3318	7.6379	0
I2C3	0	53637.9549	806613.3562	12093548.5627
I2C4	1.2101	9.9133	16.4846	0
I2C4	0	45375.1178	866980.8364	14851611.0939
I2C5	1.6918	3.2296	9.4793	0
I2C5	0	91405.5447	1718430.4179	2019771.0051
I4C0	1.0944	12.4212	13.3284	0
I4C0	0	46714.7595	670532.0143	20995190.271
I4C1	0.94632	8.0671	9.3819	0
I4C1	0	56759.0623	836038.9217	11866194.0639
I4C2	1.2539	11.0448	21.2749	0
I4C2	0	82571.2704	1834402.7913	16045431.9298
I4C3	1.3141	11.431	12.2989	0
I4C3	0	38754.9151	573242.7989	14076955.5309
I4C4	1.0208	5.9699	5.9288	0
I4C4	0	63971.5742	1347682.3612	1440100.2297
I4C5	1.3727	14.0795	19.8721	0
I4C5	0	74651.8482	933547.549	7787979.8258
I5C0	1.1724	8.4414	10.2382	0
I5C0	0	53280.5798	1204916.5266	10902065.4811
I5C1	1.1678	8.5432	9.3433	0
I5C1	0	39789.3424	634151.5786	16584598.3236
I5C2	1.1947	7.9231	11.0678	0
I5C2	0	58236.6007	1037102.2961	27012006.1519
I5C3	1.1729	7.4004	10.6367	0
I5C3	0	47127.362	982572.5208	14107894.219
I5C4	1.2079	6.9318	8.6426	0
I5C4	0	36683.3045	1047471.5022	6202264.8436
I5C5	1.1773	7.9284	10.103	0
I5C5	0	37773.7753	738290.5414	16091554.6424

A.4 Animal Trial (ch. 8)

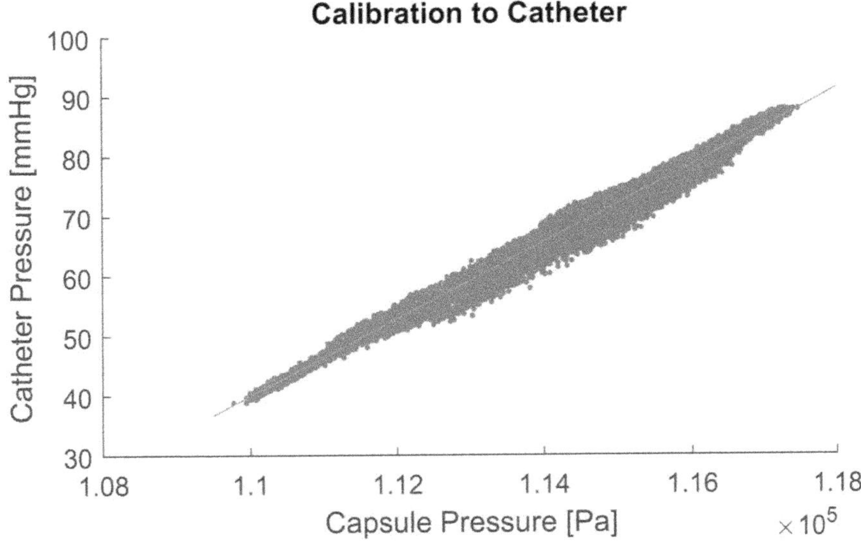

Figure A.19: Linear calibration used for the data of the 4th animal trial. Shown for sensor 0.

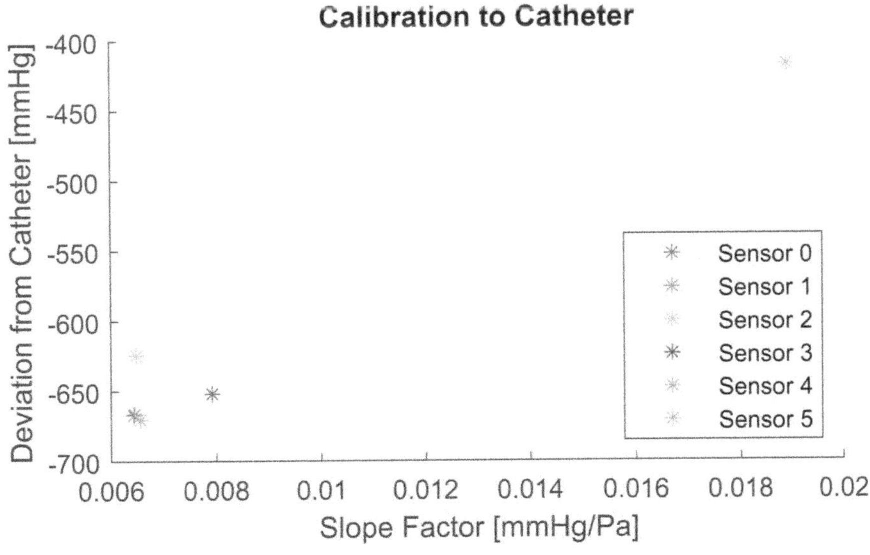

Figure A.20: Linear calibration used for the data of the 4th animal trial.

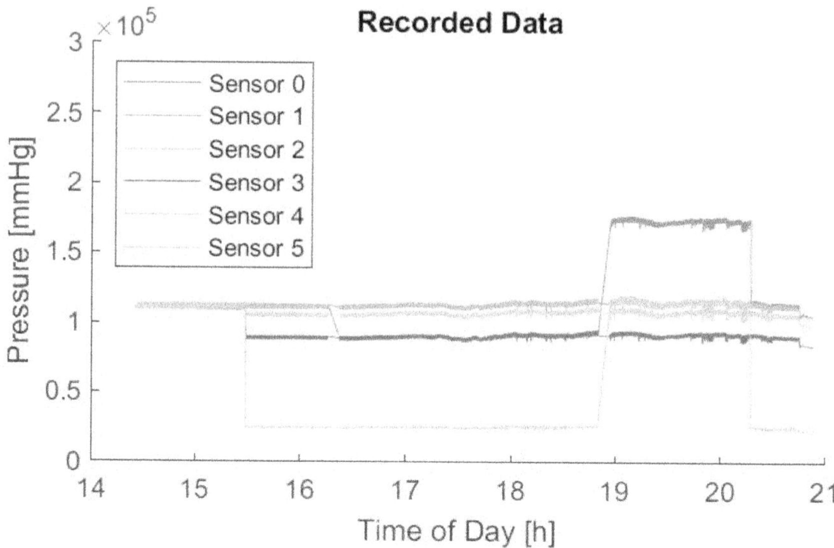

Figure A.21: Raw recorded data of the 4th animal trial showing occasional pressure jumps possibly caused by the recording software.

Table A.3: List of animal trials. Superscript refers to participated trials for the vet team lead. In Trial 1 and 2 a demonstrator was used. In all other trials Implant 4 was used.

	Date	Location	Implantation method	Outcome
Trial 1	5/22/19	FEM Berlin	single incision	ref unrecordable
Trial 2	5/29/19	FEM Berlin	single incision	ref. needle could not get a reasonable signal
Trial 3	11/3/20	FEM Remote	dual incision	ref. catheter could not get a reasonable signal
Trial 4	11/10/20	FEM Remote	dual incision	success, 2x 10 minutes of ref. signal aquired
Trial 5	10/18/21	FEM Berlin	dual incision	ref. catheter too short due to larger than usual animal
Trial 6	7/8/22	Medizin Im Gruenen	dual incision	unstable anesthesia, animal died between first and second anastomosis
Trial 7	7/8/22	Medizin Im Gruenen	dual incision	animal with damaged lung, animal died before implantation
Surgical Team	Prof. Christoph Starck, Julius Kaemmel			
Vet Team	Dr. Tanja Schmidt[1,2], Dr. Katja Reiter[3,4,5], Dr. Pia Ostach, Verena Stoessel, Dr. Juliane Unger			
Catheter	Dr. Alessio Alogna			

Bibliography

[1] M. Metra and J. R. Teerlink, "Heart failure," *Lancet*, vol. 390, no. 10106, pp. 1981–1995, 2017, doi: 10.1016/S0140-6736(17)31071-1.

[2] T. Vos, C. Allen, M. Arora, R. M. Barber, Z. A. Bhutta, A. Brown, A. Carter, D. C. Casey, F. J. Charlson, A. Z. Chen, M. Coggeshall, L. Cornaby, L. Dandona, D. J. Dicker, T. Dilegge, H. E. Erskine, A. J. Ferrari, C. Fitzmaurice, T. Fleming, M. H. Forouzanfar, N. Fullman, P. W. Gething, E. M. Goldberg, N. Graetz, J. A. Haagsma, C. O. Johnson, N. J. Kassebaum, T. Kawashima, L. Kemmer, I. A. Khalil, Y. Kinfu, H. H. Kyu, J. N. Leung, X. F. Liang, S. S. Lim, A. D. Lopez, R. Lozano, L. Marczak, G. A. Mensah, A. H. Mokdad, M. Naghavi, G. Nguyen, E. Nsoesie, H. Olsen, D. M. Pigott, C. Pinho, Z. Rankin, N. Reinig, J. A. Salomon, L. Sandar, A. Smith, J. Stanaway, C. Steiner, S. Teeple, B. A. Thomas, C. Troeger, J. A. Wagner, H. D. Wang, V. Wanga, H. A. Whiteford, L. Zoeckler, A. A. Abajobir, K. H. Abate, C. Abbafati, K. M. Abbas, F. Abd-Allah, B. Abraham, I. Abubakar, L. J. Abu-Raddad, N. M. E. Abu-Rmeileh, I. N. Ackerman, A. O. Adebiyi, Z. Ademi, A. K. Adou, K. A. Afanvi, E. E. Agardh, A. Agarwal, A. A. Kiadaliri, H. Ahmadieh, O. N. Ajala, R. O. Akinyemi, N. Akseer, Z. Al-Aly, K. Alam, N. K. M. Alam, S. F. Aldhahri, M. A. Alegretti, Z. A. Alemu, L. T. Alexander, S. Alhabib, R. Ali, A. Alkerwi, F. Alla, P. Allebeck, R. Al-Raddadi, U. Alsharif, K. A. Altirkawi, N. Alvis-Guzman, A. T. Amare, A. Amberbir *et al.*, "Global, regional, and national incidence, prevalence, and years lived with disability for 310 diseases and injuries, 1990-2015: a systematic analysis for the global burden of disease study 2015," *Lancet*, vol. 388, no. 10053, pp. 1545–1602, 2016, doi: 10.1016/s0140-6736(16)31678-6.

[3] E. J. Benjamin, P. Muntner, A. Alonso, M. S. Bittencourt, C. W. Callaway, A. P. Carson, A. M. Chamberlain, A. R. Chang, S. Cheng, S. R. Das, F. N. Delling, L. Djousse, M. S. V. Elkind, J. F. Ferguson, M. Fornage, L. C. Jordan, S. S. Khan, B. M. Kissela, K. L. Knutson, T. W. Kwan, D. T. Lackland, T. T. Lewis, J. H. Lichtman, C. T. Longenecker, M. S. Loop, P. L. Lutsey, S. S. Martin, K. Matsushita, A. E. Moran, M. E. Mussolino, M. O'Flaherty, A. Pandey, A. M. Perak, W. D. Rosamond, G. A. Roth, U. K. A. Sampson, G. M. Satou, E. B. Schroeder,

S. H. Shah, N. L. Spartano, A. Stokes, D. L. Tirschwell, C. W. Tsao, M. P. Turakhia, L. B. VanWagner, J. T. Wilkins, S. S. Wong, S. S. Virani, A. H. A. C. Epid, P. S. Comm, and S. S. Subcomm, "Heart disease and stroke statistics-2019 update a report from the american heart association," *Circulation*, vol. 139, no. 10, pp. E56–E528, 2019, doi: 10.1161/Cir.0000000000000659.

[4] G. Foster, "Third-generation ventricular assist devices," *Mechanical Circulatory and Respiratory Support*, pp. 151–186, 2018, doi: 10.1016/B978-0-12-810491-0.00005-9.

[5] V. Tchantchaleishvili, J. G. Y. Luc, C. M. Cohan, K. Phan, L. Hubbert, S. W. Day, and H. T. Masey, "Clinical implications of physiologic flow adjustment in continuous-flow left ventricular assist devices," *Asaio Journal*, vol. 63, no. 3, pp. 241–250, 2017, doi: 10.1097/Mat.0000000000000477.

[6] J. K. Kirklin, F. D. Pagani, R. L. Kormos, L. W. Stevenson, E. D. Blume, S. L. Myers, M. A. Miller, J. T. Baldwin, J. B. Young, and D. C. Naftel, "Eighth annual intermacs report: Special focus on framing the impact of adverse events," *Journal of Heart and Lung Transplantation*, vol. 36, no. 10, pp. 1080–1086, 2017, doi: 10.1016/j.healun.2017.07.005.

[7] R. F. Salamonsen, D. G. Mason, and P. J. Ayre, "Response of rotary blood pumps to changes in preload and afterload at a fixed speed setting are unphysiological when compared with the natural heart," *Artificial Organs*, vol. 35, no. 3, pp. E47–E53, 2011, doi: 10.1111/j.1525-1594.2010.01168.x.

[8] M. Vollkron, H. Schima, L. Huber, R. Benkowski, G. Morello, and G. Wieselthaler, "Development of a reliable automatic speed control system for rotary blood pumps," *Journal of Heart and Lung Transplantation*, vol. 24, no. 11, pp. 1878–1885, 2005, doi: 10.1016/j.healun.2005.02.004.

[9] D. G. Mason, A. K. Hilton, and R. F. Salamonsen, "Reliable suction detection for patients with rotary blood pumps," *Asaio Journal*, vol. 54, no. 4, pp. 359–366, 2008, doi: 10.1097/MAT.0b013e31817b5b0e.

[10] M. S. Slaughter, F. D. Pagani, J. G. Rogers, L. W. Miller, B. Sun, S. D. Russell, R. C. Starling, L. W. Chen, A. J. Boyle, S. Chillcott, R. M. Adamson, M. S. Blood, M. T. Camacho, K. A. Idrissi, M. Petty, M. Sobieski, S. Wright, T. J. Myers, D. J. Farrar, and H. I. Clinical, "Clinical management of continuous-flow left ventricular assist devices

in advanced heart failure," *Journal of Heart and Lung Transplantation*, vol. 29, no. 4, pp. S1–S39, 2010, doi: 10.1016/j.healun.2010.01.011.

[11] S. Crow, R. John, A. Boyle, S. Shumway, K. Liao, M. Colvin-Adams, C. Toninato, E. Missov, M. Pritzker, C. Martin, D. Garry, W. Thomas, and L. Joyce, "Gastrointestinal bleeding rates in recipients of nonpulsatile and pulsatile left ventricular assist devices," *J Thorac Cardiovasc Surg*, vol. 137, no. 1, pp. 208–15, 2009, doi: 10.1016/j.jtcvs.2008.07.032.

[12] S. Klotza, A. H. J. Danser, and D. Burkhoff, "Impact of left ventricular assist device (lvad) support on the cardiac reverse remodeling process," *Progress in Biophysics and Molecular Biology*, vol. 97, no. 2-3, pp. 479–496, 2008, doi: 10.1016/j.pbiomolbio.2008.02.002.

[13] I. Saito, T. Chinzei, T. Isoyama, H. Miura, A. Kouno, T. Ono, H. Nakagawa, S. Yamaguchi-Sekine, W. Shi, Y. Inoue, A. Kishi, and Y. Abe, "Implementation of the natural heartbeat synchronize control for the undulation pump ventricular assist device using the inflow pressure," *Apcmbe 2008: 7th Asian-Pacific Conference on Medical and Biological Engineering*, vol. 19, pp. 62–+, 2008, doi: 10.1007/978-3-540-79039-6_17.

[14] M. Mansouri, R. F. Salamonsen, E. Lim, R. Akmeliawati, and N. H. Lovell, "Preload-based starling-like control for rotary blood pumps: Numerical comparison with pulsatility control and constant speed operation," *PLoS One*, vol. 10, no. 4, p. e0121413, 2015, doi: 10.1371/journal.pone.0121413.

[15] A. Petrou, M. Monn, M. Meboldt, and M. S. Daners, "A novel multi-objective physiological control system for rotary left ventricular assist devices," *Annals of Biomedical Engineering*, vol. 45, no. 12, pp. 2899–2910, 2017, doi: 10.1007/s10439-017-1919-0.

[16] E. Bullister, S. Reich, and J. Sluetz, "Physiologic control algorithms for rotary blood pumps using pressure sensor input," *Artificial organs*, vol. 26, no. 11, pp. 931–938, 2002, doi: 10.1046/j.1525-1594.2002.07126.x.

[17] G. Ochsner, R. Amacher, M. J. Wilhelm, S. Vandenberghe, H. Tevaearai, A. Plass, A. Amstutz, V. Falk, and M. Schmid Daners, "A physiological controller for turbodynamic ventricular assist devices based on a measurement of the left ventricular volume," *Artificial organs*, vol. 38, no. 7, pp. 527–538, 2014, doi: 10.1111/aor.12225.

[18] Y. Wu, P. E. Allaire, G. Tao, M. Adams, Y. Liu, H. Wood, and D. B.

Olsen, "A bridge from short-term to long-term left ventricular assist device experimental verification of a physiological controller," *Artificial organs*, vol. 28, no. 10, pp. 927–932, 2004, doi: 10.1111/j.1525-1594.2004.07381.x.

[19] Y. Wu, P. E. Allaire, G. Tao, and D. Olsen, "Modeling, estimation, and control of human circulatory system with a left ventricular assist device," *IEEE transactions on control systems technology*, vol. 15, no. 4, pp. 754–767, 2007, doi: 10.1109/TCST.2006.890288.

[20] K. Ohuchi, D. Kikugawa, K. Takahashi, M. Uemura, M. Nakamura, T. Murakami, T. Sakamoto, and S. Takatani, "Control strategy for rotary blood pumps," *Artif Organs*, vol. 25, no. 5, pp. 366–70, 2001, doi: 10.1046/j.1525-1594.2001.025005366.x.

[21] A. Petrou, J. Lee, S. Dual, G. Ochsner, M. Meboldt, and M. S. Daners, "Standardized comparison of selected physiological controllers for rotary blood pumps: In vitro study," *Artificial Organs*, vol. 42, no. 3, pp. E29–E42, 2018, doi: 10.1111/aor.12999.

[22] A. Petrou, D. Kuster, J. Lee, M. Meboldt, and M. Schmid Daners, "Comparison of flow estimators for rotary blood pumps: An in vitro and in vivo study," *Ann Biomed Eng*, vol. 46, no. 12, pp. 2123–2134, 2018, doi: 10.1007/s10439-018-2106-7.

[23] A. Menditto, M. Patriarca, and B. Magnusson, "Understanding the meaning of accuracy, trueness and precision," *Accreditation and Quality Assurance*, vol. 12, no. 1, pp. 45–47, 2007, doi: 10.1007/s00769-006-0191-z.

[24] E. Bullister, S. Reich, P. d'Entremont, N. Silverman, and J. Sluetz, "A blood pressure sensor for long-term implantation," *Artificial Organs*, vol. 25, no. 5, pp. 376–379, 2001, doi: 10.1046/j.1525-1594.2001.025005376.x.

[25] B. Fritz, J. Cysyk, R. Newswanger, W. Weiss, and G. Rosenberg, "Development of an inlet pressure sensor for control in a left ventricular assist device," *Asaio Journal*, vol. 56, no. 3, pp. 180–185, 2010, doi: 10.1097/MAT.0b013e3181d2a56e.

[26] A. F. Stephens, A. Busch, R. F. Salamonsen, S. D. Gregory, and G. D. Tansley, "A novel fibre bragg grating pressure sensor for rotary ventricular assist devices," *Sensors and Actuators a-Physical*, vol. 295, pp. 474–482, 2019, doi: 10.1016/j.sna.2019.06.028.

[27] W. Shi, I. Saito, T. Chinzei, T. Isoyama, H. Miura, A. Kouno, T. Ono, H. Nakagawa, S. Yamaguchi, Y. Inoue, A. Kishi, and Y. Abe, "Development of an auto calibration method for the implantable blood pressure sensor in the undulation pump ventricular assist device (upvad)," *Apcmbe 2008: 7th Asian-Pacific Conference on Medical and Biological Engineering*, vol. 19, pp. 66–+, 2008, doi: 10.1007/978-3-540-79039-6_18.

[28] L. Brancato, G. Keulemans, T. Verbelen, B. Meyns, and R. Puers, "An implantable intravascular pressure sensor for a ventricular assist device," *Micromachines*, vol. 7, no. 8, 2016, doi: 10.3390/mi7080135.

[29] Z. X. Zhang and H. S. Dong, "A state-of-the-art overview recent development in low friction and wear-resistant coatings and surfaces for high-temperature forming tools," *Manufacturing Review*, vol. 1, 2014, doi: 10.1051/mfreview/2015001.

[30] S. Staufert and C. Hierold, "Novel sensor integration approach for blood pressure sensing in ventricular assist devices," *Proceedings of the 30th Anniversary Eurosensors Conference - Eurosensors 2016*, vol. 168, pp. 71–75, 2016, doi: 10.1016/j.proeng.2016.11.150.

[31] M. D. Zhou, C. Yang, Z. Liu, J. P. Cysyk, and S. Y. Zheng, "An implantable fabry-perot pressure sensor fabricated on left ventricular assist device for heart failure," *Biomed Microdevices*, vol. 14, no. 1, pp. 235–45, 2012, doi: 10.1007/s10544-011-9601-z.

[32] L. Hubbert, J. Baranowski, B. Delshad, and H. Ahn, "First implantation in human of a wireless miniaturized intracardiac pressure sensor in a patient with a heartmate ii (tm)," *Journal of Heart and Lung Transplantation*, vol. 33, no. 4, pp. S13–S13, 2014, doi: 10.1016/j.healun.2014.01.060.

[33] L. Hubbert, J. Baranowski, B. Delshad, and H. Ahn, "Change of left atrial pressure, lap measured with a wireless implantable pressure sensor (titan sensor) during echocardiographic ramp-test in heartmate ii patients," *Journal of Heart and Lung Transplantation*, vol. 34, no. 4, pp. S218–S219, 2015, doi: 10.1016/j.healun.2015.01.601.

[34] L. Hubbert, J. Baranowski, B. Delshad, and H. Ahn, "Left atrial pressure monitoring with an implantable wireless pressure sensor after implantation of a left ventricular assist device," *Asaio Journal*, vol. 63, no. 5, pp. E60–E65, 2017, doi: 10.1097/Mat.0000000000000451.

[35] M. Guglin, B. George, S. Branam, and A. Hart, "Cardiomems in

lvad patients: A case series," *The VAD Journal*, vol. 2, 2016, doi: 10.13023/VAD.2016.21.

[36] H. E. Verdejo, P. F. Castro, R. Concepcion, M. A. Ferrada, M. A. Alfaro, M. E. Alcaino, C. C. Deck, and R. C. Bourge, "Comparison of a radiofrequency-based wireless pressure sensor to swan-ganz catheter and echocardiography for ambulatory assessment of pulmonary artery pressure in heart failure," *Journal of the American College of Cardiology*, vol. 50, no. 25, pp. 2375–2382, 2007, doi: 10.1016/j.jacc.2007.06.061.

[37] C. Wohlgemuth, "Entwurf und galvanotechnische fertigung metallischer trennmembranen fuer mediengetrennte piezoresistive drucksensoren," Ph.D. Dissertation, Technischen Universitaet Darmstadt, 2007. [Online]. Available: http://nbn-resolving.de/urn:nbn:de:tuda-tuprints-10097

[38] V. Stankevic and C. Simkevicius, "Thermal errors in media-separating housings of pressure sensors," *Sensors and Actuators A: Physical*, vol. 75, no. 3, pp. 215–221, 1999, doi: 10.1016/S0924-4247(98)00278-7.

[39] J. C. H. Lin, P. Deng, G. Lam, B. Lu, Y. K. Lee, and Y. C. Tai, "Creep of parylene-c film," in *2011 16th International Solid-State Sensors, Actuators and Microsystems Conference*, Conference Proceedings, doi: 10.1109/TRANSDUCERS.2011.5969483. pp. 2698–2701.

[40] S. Staufert, "Conformal parylene-c media separating membranes for pressure sensing application in ventricular assist devices," Ph.D. Dissertation, ETH Zurich, 2018, doi: 10.3929/ethz-b-000346464.

[41] B. J. Kim and E. Meng, "Micromachining of parylene c for biomems," *Polymers for Advanced Technologies*, vol. 27, no. 5, pp. 564–576, 2016, doi: 10.1002/pat.3729.

[42] T. A. Harder, T. J. Yao, Q. He, C. Y. Shih, and Y. C. Tai, "Residual stress in thin-film parylene-c," *Fifteenth Ieee International Conference on Micro Electro Mechanical Systems, Technical Digest*, pp. 435–438, 2002, doi: 10.1109/Memsys.2002.984296.

[43] I. Hutter, "Leakage assessment of a parylene-c/tio2-nanostructure interface," Bachelor Thesis, ETH Zurich, 2020.

[44] R. Graf, "Optimization and miniaturization of a hermetic solder seal," Master Thesis, ETH Zurich, 2019.

[45] P. Mueller, "Miniaturization of an injection-volume optimized backside sealing," Bachelor Thesis, ETH Zurich, 2019.

[46] K. Von Petersdorff-Campen, M. A. Dupuch, K. Magkoutas, C. Hierold, and M. Schmid Daners, "Pressure and bernoulli-based flow measurement via a tapered inflow vad cannula," *IEEE Trans Biomed Eng*, vol. PP, 2021, doi: 10.1109/TBME.2021.3123983.

[47] P. Martin, "Curved membrane design and fabrication," Master Thesis, ETH Zurich, 2019.

[48] B. Mueller, "Selective tio2 nanostructure removal for parylene-c membrane fabrication," Bachelor Thesis, ETH Zurich, 2019.

Scientific Reports on Micro and Nanosystems

edited by Prof. Dr. Christofer Hierold
ETH Zürich Micro and Nanosystems

Vol. 28: Verena Maiwald, **A Microelectromechanical Switch for Bandpass Vibration Detection.**
1st Edition 2018. XVI, 164 pages. € 64,00. ISBN 978-3-86628-614-6

Vol. 29: Michelle Müller, **Micromechanical broadband vibration amplitude-amplifier for microseismic and acoustic emission detection.**
1st Edition 2019. XVIII, 168 pages. € 64,00. ISBN 978-3-86628-627-6

Vol. 30: Silvan Marc Staufert, **Conformal Parylene-C Media Separating Membranes for Pressure Sensing Applications in Ventricular Assist Devices.**
1st Edition 2019. XVIII, 150 pages. € 64,00. ISBN 978-3-86628-636-8

Vol. 31: Lalit Kumar, **Energy Dissipation, Clamping and Motional Currents in Suspended Room Temperature Carbon Nanotube Resonators.**
1st Edition 2019. XXIV, 182 pages. € 64,00. ISBN 978-3-86628-650-4

Vol. 32: Sebastian Eberle**, Ultra-clean suspended carbon nanotube gas sensors - concept for large scale fabrication and sensor characterization.**
1st Edition 2019. XX, 180 pages. € 64,00. ISBN 978-3-86628-659-7

Vol. 33: Laura Vera Jenni, **Optimization of CNT Contacts in Suspended CNTFETs and Post Dry-Transfer Processing.**
1st Edition 2019. XXII, 170 pages. € 64,00. ISBN 978-3-86628-660-3

Vol. 34: Ian Mihailovic, **Ag/BiSe memristors for sensor data storage: a novel concept for zero-power sense-log devices.**
1st Edition 2022. XXII, 146 pages. € 64,00. ISBN 978-3-86628-769-3

Vol. 35: Stefan Nedelcu, **Energy efficient analog mixed-signal front ends for CNT-FET NO2 air-quality nanosensors.**
1st Edition 2022. XVI, 232 pages. € 64,00. ISBN 978-3-86628-779-2

Vol. 36: Johannes Weichart, **Artificial Fingertip with Embedded High Resolution Tactile Sensing.**
1st Edition 2023. (10), XX, 158 pages. € 64,00. ISBN 978-3-86628-802-7

Vol. 37: Katrina Klösel, **Multifunctional materials: exploiting the versatility of Bi_2Se_3 for multimodal sensing and zero power sensor systems.**
1st Edition 2024. (8), XX, 188 pages. € 64,00. ISBN 978-3-86628-816-4

Hartung-Gorre Verlag, Konstanz http://www.hartung-gorre.de

www.ingramcontent.com/pod-product-compliance
Ingram Content Group UK Ltd.
Pitfield, Milton Keynes, MK11 3LW, UK
UKHW061826190726
13853UKWH00009B/2462